PocketGuide to Assessment in Occupational Therapy

Stanley Paul, PhD, OTR/L
Western Michigan University

David P. Orchanian, MPA, OTR, BCG
Western Michigan University

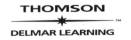

THOMSON

DELMAR LEARNING

Australia Canada Mexico Singapore Spain United Kingdom United States

THOMSON
━━━━━━━━━━━━
DELMAR LEARNING

PocketGuide to Assessment in Occupational Therapy
by
Stanley Paul, PhD, OTR/L, and David P. Orchanian, MPA, OTR, BCG

Executive Director, Health Care Business Unit: William Brottmiller

Executive Editor: Cathy L. Esperti

Developmental Editor: Juliet Byington

Editorial Assistant: Chris Manion

Executive Marketing Manager: Dawn F. Gerrain

Channel Manager: Jennifer McAvey

Art/Design Coordinator: Robert Plante

Project Editor: David Buddle

Production Coordinator: Jessica Peterson

COPYRIGHT © 2003 by Delmar Learning, a division of Thomson Learning, Inc. Thomson Learning™ is a trademark used herein under license.

Printed in the United States of America
1 2 3 4 5 XXX 07 06 05 04 03 02

For more information, contact Delmar Learning, 5 Maxwell Drive, Clifton Park, NY 12065. Or find us on the World Wide Web at http://www.delmarlearning.com

Library of Congress Cataloging-in-Publication Data
Paul, Stanley, 1964-
  PocketGuide to assessment in occupational therapy / Stanley Paul.
       p. ; cm.
Includes bibliographical references.
  ISBN 0-7668-3628-2
  1. Occupational therapy—Handbooks, manuals, etc. 2.
Diagnosis—Handbooks, manuals, etc.
  [DNLM: 1. Occupational Therapy—Handbooks. WB 39 P324p 2003] I.
Title: Pocket guide to assessment in occupational therapy. II.
Orchanian, David P. III. Title.
  RM735.3 .P38 2003
  615.8'515—dc21

                                            2002013369

Notice to the Reader

Contents

v

Preface

This *PocketGuide to Assessment in Occupational Therapy* is a quick reference for developing and planning assessment strategies for occupational therapy students, instructors, and clinicians. The clear, easy-to-follow format provides applicable information on a variety of conditions frequently encountered in the domain of occupational therapy. The assessments suggested are not intended to be all-inclusive; rather, the authors have provided a representative sample of assessments—both formal and informal—that may be relevant to a given client and condition. It is essential to understand that the assessment process is a dynamic event or series of events. Client assessment and reassessment is ongoing from the time clinical services are initiated to the date of service discontinuation or discharge, and this pocketguide is a tool to aid in that process of assessment.

In using this pocketguide, it is important that the reader understand what is good assessment:

- It is individually designed to address the needs and expectations of the client. The occupational therapist and client should collaborate in order to plan and implement an assessment strategy that is client-centered and will also provide relevant information to the treatment team.
- It is holistic, recognizing the physical, psychosocial, emotional, cultural, and financial factors that may have bearing on function and functional performance. The occupational therapist who is administering a standardized cognitive assessment should also be considering performance components such as motor control, postural control, strength, and dexterity.
- It is understood by the client, his family, and other members of the interdisciplinary team.
- The assessment is readily administered and interpreted by a wide range of clinicians from entry level to those with vast clinical or academic experience.

The advantages of accurate and effective assessing include:

- Helps to define client concerns. What are clients having trouble doing?
- Focuses on the present. An easy starting point for exploring possible etiologies.
- Measures client's ability to function despite disease or disability.

- Identifies client's strengths and resources available to alleviate or minimize deficits.
- Promotes realistic, client-focused goal setting.

To perform assessments effectively, specialized skills and competence are required including:

- Interviewing skills.
- Ability to establish and maintain empathic relationships.
- Experience conducting health and social assessments.
- Knowledge of human behavior, family and caregiver dynamics, life span development, disability.
- Awareness of community resources and services.

How the PocketGuide Is Organized

The *PocketGuide to Assessment in Occupational Therapy* is organized around the major disabilities that occupational therapists encounter in their everyday practice. These include physical, psychosocial, geriatric, pediatric, and developmental diagnoses. Assessment guidelines are developed for the major disabilities. Additionally, there are brief summaries for each condition addressing such areas as: etiology, symptoms, and prognosis/outcomes. Each main condition contains information related to assessment objectives, assessment of performance areas, assessment of performance components, and suggested standardized assessments and tools relevant to the specific condition.

Each condition is printed in blue text and each cross-referenced entry is underlined in blue to indicate that there is a complete entry on that topic. Conditions are listed alphabetically with subcategories of a given disorder described under the main entry. All references are located in the back of the text, along with a glossary and related appendices.

The appendices include a list of commonly used acronyms contained in the text, information on home evaluation as an assessment intervention, a list of assessments and related contact information including a brief statement of purpose for each assessment listed, and web addresses of health organizations.

AIDS See <u>human immunodeficiency virus</u>.

Alzheimer's disease

Alzheimer's disease is an irreversible, progressive process that destroys neuronal structures in the brain, resulting in declines in memory, performance of routine tasks, time and space orientation, language and communication skills, abstract thinking, and the ability to learn and carry out mathematical calculations (National Institute on Aging, 1995). Of the population exhibiting symptoms of dementia, approximately half are thought to have dementia of the Alzheimer's type (National Institute on Aging, 1995). Alzheimer's disease is a diagnosis by exclusion, meaning all other possible reasons must be ruled out before the diagnosis of Alzheimer's disease or senile dementia of the Alzheimer's type (SDAT) is applied.

Etiology

The most definitive way to diagnose Alzheimer's disease is by observing characteristic neuritic plaques and neurofibrillary tangles during brain autopsy. Plaques and tangles interfere with the affected neurons' ability to synapse with other neurons, and they may even die. Neurotransmission is further impaired as a result of a lack of acetylcholine, which is critical for memory and has been found to drop by 90% in individuals with Alzheimer's disease (National Institute on Aging, 1995). Studies indicate that dementia of the Alzheimer's type may have many causes, including genetic, environmental, traumatic, viral, and metabolic factors.

Symptoms

The *DSM-IV* requires the following criteria for a diagnosis of dementia of the Alzheimer's type, the development of multiple cognitive deficits manifested by other memory impairment, and one or more of the following cognitive disturbances: aphasia, apraxia, agnosia, or disturbance in executive functioning such as planning, organizing, sequencing, or abstracting. The cognitive deficits cause significant impairment in social or occupational functioning and represent a significant decline from a previous level of function. The course is characterized by gradual onset and continuing cognitive decline. The cognitive deficits are not caused by central nervous system disorders, systemic conditions, substance-induced conditions, or other mental illness.

Assessment Objectives

The OT will be responsible for assessing occupational performance areas and components. All areas assessed will be considered in relation to functional performance. Key areas for assessment include various performance areas and skills in order to identify realistic client-centered treatment goals.

Assessment of Performance Areas

- Activities of daily living: BADLs and IADLs
- Work and productive activities: Homemaking skills and use of assistive devices
- Play and leisure activities

Assessment of Performance Components

Sensory Processing

- Tactile
- Proprioceptive
- Vestibular
- Visual

Neuromusculoskeletal

- Postural control and balance
- Mobility
- Motor planning

Perceptual Processing

- Spatial relations
- Kinesthesis
- Right-left discrimination
- Position in space
- Depth perception

Cognitive Integration and Cognitive Components

- Executive skills (IADLs)
- Orientation
- Memory (recent and remote)
- Attention span
- Safety and judgment

Psychosocial Skills

- Social interaction

Standardized Assessment Tools

- Mini Mental State Exam (MMSE)
- Middlesex Elderly Assessment of Mental State (MEAMS)

- The Cognitive Assessment of Minnesota (CAM)
- Kohlman Evaluation of Living Skills (KELS)
- Allen Cognitive Level Scale (ACLS)
- Assessment of Motor and Process Skills (AMPS)
- Functional Independence Measure (FIM^{SM})

Other Tools
- Home safety evaluation

Prognosis and Outcome

Progressive loss of cognitive functions is generally to be expected. Physical body systems may remain in relatively good health for a significant period of time after the onset of cognitive decline. Positive functional outcomes in areas of self-care and leisure can be expected in the early stage of the disease. In advanced and terminal stages, loss of functional skills is unavoidable.

amputation

Amputation refers to removal of part of a body segment. Peripheral vascular disease, with or without diabetes, is the leading cause of amputation in the United States. Other causes of amputation may include trauma, burns, surgical intervention, or cancer.

Etiology

The two most common causes of amputation in the upper extremity are trauma and surgical removal. Trauma such as tearing, laceration, burns, and crushing injuries comprise the majority of injuries resulting in amputation. Common diseases that lead to amputation are peripheral vascular disease and diabetes mellitus, with resultant loss of portions of the lower extremity. Specific premorbid health factors tend to increase the potential for eventual loss of a limb, including duration and management of diabetes, history of leg, foot, or toe ulcers and/or injuries, hypertension, and smoking.

Symptoms

There is not one consistent classification system and set of terms used to describe the site of amputation. Most classification systems use the level of amputation as a descriptor, with variation based upon whether the bone or joint is used as the reference point (e.g., transradial vs. below elbow). Several classification systems mix reference to a bone or a joint (Rock, 1996; Morris & Muhn, 1998). See classification by level below:

- Partial hand
- Wrist disarticulation
- Long below-elbow
- Short below-elbow
- Elbow disarticulation
- Long above-elbow
- Short above-elbow
- Shoulder disarticulation
- Forequarter

Assessment Objectives

The occupational therapist will be involved in the assessment and management of the amputee from the preoperative stage to discharge home and into the community. The OT assists the patient in identifying his or her own goals and those occupational roles that are relevant and important to the client. All basic activities of daily living (BADLs) are assessed. In some cases it will be beneficial to assess instrumental activities of daily living (IADLs), such as meal planning, check-writing, budgeting, using public transportation, and developing community mobility skills. Work, education, and leisure activities may also be assessed.

Assessment of Performance Areas

- Activities of Daily Living: BADLs and IADLs
- Work and Productive Activities: Homemaking skills, adaptive work techniques, energy conservation, and use of assistive devices and technology
- Play and leisure activities

Assessment of Performance Components

Sensory Processing
- Tactile
- Proprioceptive

Perceptual Processing
- Kinesthesia
- Pain response
- Body scheme
- Position in space

Neuromusculoskeletal
- Range of motion (PROM and AROM)
- Muscle tone

- Strength
- Endurance
- Postural control
- Soft tissue integrity

Motor
- Gross coordination
- Bilateral integration
- Motor control

Cognitive Integration
- Attention span
- Problem solving
- Learning and generalization

Psychosocial Skills
- Interests
- Self-concept
- Role performance, coping skills

Home Assessment

Factors of importance to consider in the home assessment include:

- Home safety
- Assistive devices and equipment
- Home modification
- Exterior access
- Ramping

Standardized Assessment Tools

- Functional Independence Measure (FIM^{SM})
- Functional Independence Measure for Children (Wee FIM^{SM})
- Barthel Index
- Modified Interest Checklist
- Self-Esteem Scale
- Worker Role Inventory
- Assessment of Motor and Process Skills (AMPS)
- Verbal Rating Scale
- Numeric Rating Scale
- Tennessee Self-Concept Scale—Revised (TSCS)

Other Tools
- Manual Muscle Test (MMT)
- Range of Motion Test (AROM/PROM)

- Goniometer
- Dynamometer

Prognosis and Outcome

Positive outcome for the proper healing of the residual limb, prosthetic fitting, and rehabilitation with the prosthesis requires:

- Cognitive skills
- Motivation
- Effective training
- Proper care and maintenance of the prosthesis
- Management of underlying disease or condition causing the amputation

amyotrophic lateral sclerosis

Amyotrophic lateral sclerosis (ALS) is a fatal neuromuscular disease characterized by progressive muscle weakness resulting in paralysis.

Etiology

At least 10% of ALS cases are hereditary. This is called familial ALS. Generally, familial ALS is defined as two or more cases in the same bloodline. In familial ALS the disease is autosomal dominant, meaning that if a parent has ALS, their children have a 50% chance of inheriting the defective gene. While the risk of inheriting the defective gene is 50% for each child of an affected person, not all people with the defective gene will develop the disorder. Ninety percent of ALS cases have no familial link; these are called sporadic ALS.

Symptoms

ALS symptoms may include tripping, stumbling and falling, loss of muscle control and strength in the hands and arms, difficulty speaking, swallowing and/or breathing, chronic fatigue, and muscle twitching and/or cramping. ALS is characterized by both upper and lower motor neuron damage. Symptoms of upper motor neuron damage include stiffness (spasticity), muscle twitching (fasciculations), and muscle shaking (clonus). Symptoms of lower motor neuron damage include muscle weakness and muscle shrinking (atrophy).

Assessment Objectives

The occupational therapist will be responsible for assessing occupational performance areas and components. All areas assessed

6

will be considered in relation to functional performance. Key areas for assessment include various performance areas and skills in order to identify realistic client-centered treatment goals.

Assessment of Performance Areas

- Activities of Daily Living: BADLs and IADLs
- Work and Productive Activities: Homemaking, adaptive work techniques, energy conservation, and use of assistive devices and technology
- Leisure Activities

Assessment of Performance Components

Sensory Processing
- Tactile
- Proprioceptive

Perceptual Processing
- Stereognosis
- Kinesthesia
- Position in space

Neuromusculoskeletal
- Reflex
- Range of motion
- Muscle tone
- Strength
- Endurance
- Postural control
- Postural alignment
- Soft tissue integrity

Motor
- Gross coordination
- Bilateral integration
- Motor control
- Fine coordination/dexterity
- Oral-motor control

Cognitive Integration
- Level of arousal
- Attention span
- Problem solving
- Generalization

Psychosocial
- Interests
- Self-concept
- Role performance
- Coping skills

Standardized Assessment Tools

- Barthel Index
- Katz Index of ADL
- Functional Independence Measure (FIM^{SM})
- Tinetti Test of Balance
- Berg Test of Balance
- Role Checklist
- Dysphagia Evaluation Protocol
- Verbal Rating Scale (Verbal Descriptor Scale)
- The Pain Estimate (Numeric Rating Scale)
- Visual Analogue Pain Rating Scale
- The Cognitive Assessment of Minnesota (CAM)
- Mini Mental Status Exam (MMSE)
- Geriatric Depression Screen (GDS)
- Self-Esteem Scale
- Tennessee Self-Concept Scale—Revised (TSCS)

Other Tools
- Grip strength test
- Pinch test
- Jamar dynamometer
- Goniometer
- Range of motion test (AROM/PROM)

Prognosis and Outcome

ALS is almost always fatal. There are rare cases where the disease progression plateaus or stops. There are a few cases of people reporting a reversal of symptoms. If an ALS client opts for a ventilator, he or she can live for many years with the disease.

The primary desired outcome is to maximize and maintain ADL function and to reduce dependence on caregivers for as long as feasible. Incorporation of assistive devices and environmental adaptations can aid client and caregiver in achieving maximized levels of function and quality of life.

anorexia nervosa See eating disorders.

arthritis See osteoarthritis and rheumatoid arthritis.

arthrogryposis multiplex congenita

Arthrogryposis multiplex congenita (AMC) is a musculoskeletal disorder characterized by the presence of multiple joint contractures at birth. In some cases, only a few joints may be affected; however, in the classic cases of AMC, hands, wrists, elbows, shoulders, hips, feet, and knees are affected. In the more severe cases, joints in the back can be affected as well. In addition to having joint contractures, children also experience muscle weakness, which further limits movement (Tomcheck, 1999).

Etiology

There are as many as 10 to 20 different arthrogrypotic disorders, all with similar joint manifestations. The most common form of AMC is amyoplasia. There are many different causes of AMC, but typically it is the result of either problems with joint growth and development, decreased fetal movement (not enough room in the uterus to move), or problems with spinal development in the first three months of pregnancy. AMC occurs in 1 out of every 3,000 live births. In most cases, AMC is not inherited and does not occur more than once in a family. However, in about 30% of the cases, a genetic cause has been identified.

Symptoms

A diagnosis of AMC can sometimes be made during pregnancy; ultrasounds at approximately 20 weeks' gestation may show abnormal position of joints or lack of movements in joints and limbs, indicating the disorder. Otherwise, the diagnosis can be made by an orthopedist based on clinical symptoms and findings. The following features can be seen in some children with AMC:

- Normal intelligence
- Intact sensation
- Muscle weakness
- Internal rotation deformity of the shoulder
- Extension and pronation deformity of the elbow
- Volar and ulnar deformity of the wrist
- Finger in fixed flexion and thumb-in-palm deformity

- Flexed, abducted, externally rotated hips, often with dislocation
- Flexion deformity of the knee
- Clubfoot deformity

Assessment Objectives

The occupational therapist will be responsible for assessing occupational performance areas and components. All areas assessed will be considered in relation to functional performance. Key areas for assessment include various performance areas and skills in order to identify realistic client-centered treatment goals.

Assessment of Performance Areas

- Activities of daily living: BADL and IADL skills
- Work and productive areas: educational and vocational activities
- Play/leisure activities

Assessment of Performance Components

Sensory Processing
- Tactile
- Proprioceptive
- Vestibular
- Visual

Perceptual Processing
- Stereognosis
- Kinesthesia
- Pain response
- Body scheme
- Position in space
- Topographical orientation

Neuromusculoskeletal
- Reflex
- Range of motion
- Muscle tone
- Strength
- Endurance
- Postural control
- Postural alignment
- Soft tissue integrity

Motor
- Gross coordination
- Crossing the midline

- Laterality
- Bilateral integration
- Motor control
- Praxis
- Fine coordination/dexterity

Cognitive Integration and Cognitive Components

- Attention span
- Initiation of activity
- Termination of activity
- Memory and sequencing
- Spatial operations
- Problem solving
- Learning
- Generalization

Psychosocial Skills

- Interests
- Self-concept
- Social conduct
- Interpersonal skills
- Self-expression
- Coping

Standardized Assessment Tools

- Battelle Developmental Inventory (BDI)
- Movement Assessment of Infants (MAI)
- Toddler and Infant Motor Evaluation (TIME)
- Vineland Adaptive Behavior Scales-Revised (VABS-R)
- Clinical Observations of Motor and Postural Skills (COMPS)
- WeeFIM℠ Version 4.0

Other Tools

- Manual Muscle Test (MMT)
- Range of Motion Test (PROM/AROM)
- Goniometer
- Dynamometer
- Pinch/Grip Meter

Prognosis and Outcome

There is no cure for AMC. There are treatments that can assist children in living full and productive lives. Physical therapy and occupational therapy have proven to be beneficial to strengthening muscles and maximizing active and passive range of motion. Splinting and the use of orthotics can also assist in maintaining range of motion. In the event that these traditional approaches do not produce positive results, surgery may be necessary. In some cases muscle and tendon transfers can be done to improve range of motion. Fortunately, AMC is not a progressive disorder, so it will not worsen with age. It is essential that children receive proper assessment and treatment to prevent joints from stiffening as they grow. Most children with AMC have some ability to ambulate. Bracing and other interventions aid ambulation. AMC may be accompanied by other disorders, such as a central nervous system disorder, but the long-term outlook is generally positive. Most individuals with AMC are of normal intelligence and are able to lead productive lives.

athletic injuries, sports injuries

Athletic injuries are incurred during participation in competitive or noncompetitive sports or during training sessions. Sports may include baseball, football, hockey, golf, gymnastics, rock climbing, tennis, skiing, volleyball, weightlifting, and many others. More than 10 million sports injuries are treated each year in the United States (Laskowski, 1996). The principles of sports medicine can be applied to the treatment of many musculoskeletal injuries, which resemble athletic injuries but have different causes. For example, tennis elbow can be caused by carrying a suitcase, turning a screw, or opening a stuck door, and runner's knee can be caused by excessive inward rolling of the foot (pronation) while walking. Most musculoskeletal injuries can be divided into two broad categories—acute and subacute, or chronic. Acute injuries are often related to a breach of integrity of the muscular system, such as a bone fracture or ligamentous disruption. The range of severity is broad and includes everything from a mild inversion ankle sprain to a devastating spinal cord injury.

The basic principles of rehabilitation after musculoskeletal injury include pain reduction by means of various modalities (i.e., ice, superficial and deep heat, interferential current) and appropriately prescribed medications, splinting, restoration of range of motion and flexibility, therapeutic strengthening, maximization of sport-specific agility, coordination, and proprioception before return to sports (Laskowski, 1996). The following is a list of the common athletic injuries to the upper extremity:

Shoulder
- Shoulder separation
- Tendinitis
- Bursitis
- Impingement syndrome
- Torn rotator cuff
- Frozen shoulder (adhesive capsulitis)
- Shoulder fracture
- Arthritis of the shoulder
- Joint noise, pops and cracks
- Muscle sprains and strains

Elbow
- Lateral epicondylitis or tennis elbow
- Medial epicondylitis or golfer's elbow
- Triceps tendinitis
- Elbow dislocation
- Bursitis of the elbow
- Fracture of the head of the radius

Forearm
- Radial tunnel syndrome
- Pronator syndrome

Wrist and Hand
- Tendinitis of the wrist
- de Quervain's syndrome
- Carpal tunnel syndrome
- Guyon's canal syndrome or "handlebar palsy"
- Ulnar collateral ligament injury (skier's or gamekeeper's thumb)
- Fracture of the thumb
- Finger fractures
- Dislocations at interphalangeal joints
- Boutonniere deformity
- Mallet finger
- Muscle sprains and strains

Etiology

Athletic injuries are caused by faulty training methods, structural abnormalities that stress certain parts of the body more than others, and weakness of muscles, tendons, and ligaments. Injuries occur as a result of high-speed objects or external forces impacting on the upper extremity and producing contusions or shearing or repetitive stress. Many of these injuries are caused by chronic wear and tear, which results from repetitive motion stressing susceptible tissue.

Symptoms

The primary symptoms of athletic injuries are:

- Change in posture of the extremity or part involved in the injury
- Pain, including numbness and tingling
- Edema
- Inability to move the extremity or part injured
- Limitations in joint range, lack of joint mobility or flexibility
- Muscle weakness
- Loss of sensation—touch, pressure, localization and proprioception, temperature and vibration, stereognosis
- Hand function deficits—grip, grasp, manipulation, dexterity and bilateral coordination
- Skin changes—color and condition

Assessment Objectives

The OT will be responsible for assessing occupational performance areas and components. Evaluation and treatment of the athlete with an upper extremity injury should be safe and effective with a keen awareness of the possible return of the athlete to the sport. All areas assessed will be considered in relation to functional performance. Key areas for assessment include various performance areas and skills in order to identify realistic client-centered treatment goals.

Assessment of Performance Areas

- Activities of daily living: BADL and simple IADL skills
- Play and leisure skills
- School/educational setting if applicable
- Work/productivity skills

Assessment of Performance Components

Sensory Processing
- Proprioceptive
- Tactile

Perceptual Processing
- Stereognosis
- Kinesthesia
- Pain response
- Position in space

Neuromusculoskeletal
- Reflex
- Range of motion
- Muscle tone
- Strength
- Endurance
- Soft tissue integrity

Motor
- Gross coordination
- Bilateral integration
- Motor control
- Fine coordination/dexterity

Cognitive Integration
- Problem solving
- Learning
- Generalization

Psychosocial Skills/Psychological Components
- Values
- Interests
- Role performance
- Social conduct
- Coping skills

Standardized Assessment Tools

- Goniometer, dynamometer, pinch meter
- Circumferential or volumetric measurement of edema
- Manual muscle test
- Hand function test
- Sensory testing
- ADL scales

- Home and environmental evaluation
- Occupational performance history
- Leisure activities checklist

Standardized Tests
- Functional Independence Measure (FIM^{SM})
- Barthel Index
- Minnesota Rate of Manipulation Test (MRMT)
- Minnesota Manual Dexterity Test (MMDT)
- Jebson Hand Function Test
- Purdue Pegboard
- McGill Pain Questionnaire (MPQ)
- Modified Interest Checklist
- Occupational Performance History Interview
- Worker Role Interview

Prognosis and Outcome

Prognosis varies depending on the severity of the injury, intensity of rehabilitation therapy, and limitations presented by coexisting medical diagnoses. The outcome of therapy also depends on the cognition, learning skills, and motivation of the individual, notably in hand function re-education programs. Usually the conditions improve with medical and surgical intervention, hand therapy supplemented and continued with home program, splinting, and activity modifications. Complete recovery to normalcy may not be achievable in all cases.

attention deficit/hyperactive disorder

Attention deficit hyperactive disorder (ADHD), also known as minimal brain dysfunction, hyperkinetic impulse disorder, and hyperactive child syndrome, involves a persistent and frequent pattern of developmentally inappropriate inattention and impulsivity with or without hyperactivity (*DSM-IV*). The *Diagnostic and Statistical Manual,* 4th Edition (*DSM-IV*) identifies three types of ADHD: Predominantly Hyperactive-Impulsive Type, Predominantly Inattentive Type, and Combined Type. ADHD is seen in both children and adults. According to the American Psychiatric Association, it is estimated that there are approximately 1.6 to 2 million people who have this disorder (*DSM-IV*). Boys are more commonly affected than girls are by a 10:1 ratio. ADHD influences the behavior of a child at any cognitive level except for moderate to profound mental retardation. Children with ADHD are not unable to learn, but they do have difficulty performing in school due to poor organization, inattention, and distractibility. Some children with ADHD also have learning disabilities, which additionally complicate identification and treatment. Children with ADHD are guaranteed a free and appropriate education to meet their needs under two federal laws: the Individuals with Disabilities Education Act of 1990, and Section 504 of the Rehabilitation Act of 1973 (Office for Civil Rights, 1988).

Etiology

The cause is unknown. Several theories advocating biochemical, sensorimotor, physiologic, and behavioral correlates and manifestations have been proposed. Although we do not know from what specific parts of the brain ADHD arises, current hypotheses associate it with abnormalities of connections in the outermost layer at the front of the brain; it may involve faulty regulation of certain brain chemical messenger systems, predominantly those that use dopamine and norepinephrine (Biederman & Faraone, 1996).

Other hypotheses include effects of toxins, neurologic immaturity, infections, drug exposure in utero, head injuries, and environmental factors (Beers & Berkow, 1999).

Symptoms

To meet the diagnostic criteria for ADHD, symptoms must be evident for at least 6 months, with onset before the age of seven and in two or more settings (school, work, and home). There must be clear evidence of clinically significant impairment in social, academic, or occupational functioning. Diagnostic criteria/symptoms are listed below.

Inattention
- Often fails to give close attention to details or makes careless mistakes in schoolwork, work, or other activities
- Often has difficulty sustaining attention in tasks or play activities
- Often does not seem to listen when spoken to directly
- Often does not follow through on instructions and fails to finish schoolwork, chores, or duties in the workplace (not due to oppositional behavior or failure to understand instructions)

- Often has difficulty organizing tasks and activities
- Often avoids, dislikes, or is reluctant to engage in tasks that require sustained mental effort (such as schoolwork or home-work)
- Often loses things necessary for tasks or activities (e.g., toys, school assignments, pencils, books, or tools)
- Is often easily distracted by extraneous stimuli
- Is often forgetful in daily activities

Hyperactivity-Impulsivity

- Often fidgets with hands or feet or squirms in seat
- Often leaves seat in classroom or in other situations in which remaining seated is expected
- Often runs about or climbs excessively in situations in which it is inappropriate (in adolescents or adults, may be limited to subjective feelings of restlessness)
- Often has difficulty playing or engaging in leisure activities quietly
- Is often "on the go" or often acts as if "driven by a motor"
- Often talks excessively
- Often blurts out answers before questions have been com-pleted
- Often has difficulty awaiting turn
- Often interrupts or intrudes on others

Assessment Objectives

The occupational therapist will be responsible for assessing occupational performance areas and components. All areas assessed will be considered in relation to functional performance. Key areas for assessment include various performance areas and skills in order to identify realistic client-centered treatment goals.

Assessment of Performance Areas

- Activities of daily living: BADL and simple IADL skills
- Play and leisure skills
- School/educational setting if applicable
- Work/productivity skills

Assessment of Performance Components

Sensory Processing

- Proprioceptive
- Tactile

- Vestibular
- Visual
- Auditory
- Gustatory
- Olfactory

Perceptual Processing
- Stereognosis
- Kinesthesia
- Position in space
- Body scheme
- Right-left discrimination
- Depth perception
- Spatial relations
- Topographical orientation

Neuromusculoskeletal
- Range of motion
- Muscle tone
- Strength
- Endurance

Motor
- Gross coordination
- Bilateral integration
- Motor control
- Praxis
- Fine coordination/dexterity
- Laterality
- Crossing the midline
- Visual-motor integration
- Oral-motor control

Cognitive Integration
- Level of arousal
- Attention span
- Memory
- Initiation of activity
- Termination of activity
- Problem solving
- Sequencing
- Spatial operations

- Learning
- Generalization

Psychosocial Skills/Psychological Components

- Values
- Interests
- Self-concept
- Role performance
- Social conduct
- Coping skills
- Self-control
- Time management

Standardized Assessment Tools

Assessment Tools

- ADL scales
- Developmental scales
- Hand function tests
- Play scales
- Prevocational skill testing for adults and young adults
- Cognitive and perceptual tests

Standardized Tests

- Sensory Integration and Praxis Tests (SIPT)
- Sensory Profile
- Developmental Test of Visual Perception, 2nd Edition (DTVP-2)
- Children's Playfulness Scale
- Play Observation
- Peabody Developmental Motor Scales (PDMS)
- Bayley Scales of Infant Development-II (BSID-II)
- Functional Independence Measure (FIM^{SM}) and Functional Independence Measure for Children (Wee FIM^{SM})
- Vineland Adaptive Behavior Scales-Revised (VABS-R)

Prognosis and Outcome

Attention deficit/hyperactive disorder is a lifelong condition. Attention deficit disorder that lasts into adulthood is referred to as ADD-RT (Residual Type). Thirty to eighty percent of children with ADHD persist into adolescence. Sixty-five percent of adolescent ADHD persists into adulthood. Poor prognosis is predicted by low IQ, adult-directed oppositional and aggressive behavior, and poor peer relations. Compensatory learned techniques will be required with periodic modification as the individual grows.

autism

Autism is a disorder that manifests between the ages of 0 and 3 years with impaired social development, communication skills, and lack of interest in activities (American Psychiatric Association, 1994). There are two types based on its clinical onset. In the first type the symptoms appear soon after birth. In the second type the child develops normally until 1 to 2 years and then regresses, losing acquired social and communication skills.

Etiology

The cause of autism in unknown but there are a number of theories suggesting possible causes. Theories suggest autism is a neurological disorder affecting the neuroanatomy and neurochemistry of the brain. Magnetic resonance imaging (MRI) has identified hypoplasia of the cerebellar vermis. Other suggested causes include cytomegalic inclusion disorder, congenital rubella syndrome, phenylketonuria, and fragile X syndrome (American Psychiatric Association, 1994; Cammisa & Hobbs, 1993). The male to female incident ratio is 4:1 and it occurs in approximately 4 out of 10,000 births.

Symptoms

ADL, Play, and Leisure

- Delay of normal developmental milestones
- Difficulty transferring learning from lower skills to more advanced skills
- Lack of social development to appropriate age level, lack of social play skills, and tendency for solitary play
- Lack of interest and curiosity about social events

Sensorimotor

- Ritual behaviors or self-stimulating behaviors such as stereotypy and repetitive mannerisms such as body rocking, spinning, finger flapping, head banging, or other complex movements
- May refuse to hold objects
- May exhibit decreased muscle tone and inadequate postural control

- May tend to avoid activities that need physical exertion
- May have poor spatial relationships
- May have sensory processing disorder
- May avoid eye gaze
- May have poor motor planning

Cognitive
- Preoccupation with stereotypical events and patterns
- Learning disorder
- Poor attention span and orientation
- Lack of eye contact
- Inability to form novel concepts
- Good rote memory and special skills such as doing puzzles, musical ability, and memorizing details
- Inability to make transition from one activity to another

Psychosocial
- Impairment of nonverbal communication skills and social gestures
- Lack of interest in family members
- Delayed spoken language
- Lack of awareness about others' feelings
- Fails to cuddle when held and strong attachment to objects
- Does not show distress when separated from parent or caregiver
- Inability to imitate social behaviors

Environmental
- Resistance to change in the environment
- Inflexible adherence to nonfunctional routines and rituals

Assessment Objectives

The OT will be responsible for assessing occupational performance areas and components, social skills, and development. All areas assessed will be considered in relation to functional performance. Key areas for assessment include various performance areas and skills in order to identify realistic client-centered treatment goals.

Assessment of Performance Areas

- Activities of daily living: BADL and simple IADL skills
- Play and leisure skills

- Work/productivity history and prevocational skills need to be evaluated in older children and adults

Assessment of Performance Components

Sensory Processing
- Proprioceptive
- Tactile
- Vestibular
- Visual
- Auditory
- Gustatory
- Olfactory

Perceptual Processing
- Stereognosis
- Kinesthesia
- Position in space
- Body scheme
- Right-left discrimination
- Depth perception
- Spatial relations
- Topographical orientation

Neuromusculoskeletal
- Range of motion
- Muscle tone
- Strength
- Endurance
- Postural control

Motor
- Gross coordination
- Bilateral integration
- Motor control
- Praxis
- Fine coordination/dexterity
- Laterality
- Crossing the midline
- Visual-motor integration
- Oral-motor control

Cognitive Integration
- Level of arousal
- Orientation
- Recognition
- Attention span
- Memory
- Initiation of activity
- Termination of activity
- Problem solving
- Sequencing
- Spatial operations
- Concept formation
- Learning
- Generalization

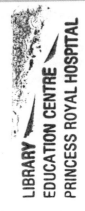

Psychosocial Skills/Psychological Components
- Interests
- Self-concept
- Role performance
- Social conduct
- Interpersonal skills
- Coping skills
- Self-control
- Time management

Standardized Assessment Tools

- ADL scales
- Developmental scales
- Hand function test
- Play scales
- Prevocational skill testing for adults and young adults
- Sensorimotor scales
- Cognitive and perceptual tests

Standardized Tests
- Sensory Integration and Praxis Tests (SIPT)
- Sensory Profile
- Children's Playfulness Scale
- Play Observation
- Bayley Scales of Infant Development-II (BSID-II)
- Vineland Adaptive Behavior Scales-Revised (VABS-R)

Prognosis and Outcome

Prognosis is dependent on the chronicity of the disorder. Often a person may be able to function semi-independently at home or group homes. Individuals with chronic autistic disorder may need highly structured environments such as nursing homes or hospitals. A person might be able to become independent in simple ADL and leisure skills. A person with mild involvement might be able to learn some social, coping, and work skills.

battle fatigue syndrome See <u>post traumatic stress disorder</u>.

blindness See <u>low vision</u>.

brachial plexus injury

Brachial plexus injuries, also referred to as Erb's palsy, Klumpke's palsy, and Erb-Duchenne-Klumpke palsy, produce a mixed motor and sensory disorder in the corresponding limb. Injury or dysfunction in the brachial plexus does not fit the distribution of individual roots or nerves. The brachial plexus forms from the ventral rami of spinal roots C5 to T1. Brachial plexus lesions have been classified as supraclavicular (upper plexus) or infraclavicular (lower plexus) lesions. They are also characterized by cause or as complete or incomplete. Disorders of the rostral (upper) brachial plexus (C5, 6) produce disability about the shoulder and elbow, and those of the caudal (lower) brachial plexus produce disability in the forearm, wrist, and hand.

Detailed knowledge of plexus anatomy is crucial in assessment of brachial plexus disorders. Electromyography is the only technological means of determining plexus function. Electrodiagnostic evaluation is done to locate the lesion, characterize the pathophysiology, and to establish the prognosis and treatment plan.

Etiology

The most common causes of brachial plexus injury are stretch injury due to excessive limb excursion (traction), compression by neighboring structures, and iatrogenic insults. Contusion or penetration in utero may also cause brachial plexus injuries. Radiation treatment for <u>cancer</u> can cause radiation induced brachial plexopathy. In adults, the most common causes are trauma resulting from fractures of the clavicle or humerus, subluxation of the shoulder or cervical spine, or metastatic cancer invasion into the surrounding areas.

Symptoms

In upper brachial plexus disorders, the muscles affected are rhomboids, serratus anterior, supraspinatus, infraspinatus, pectoralis major (sternoclavicular portion), biceps, flexor carpi radialis, latissimus dorsi, subscapularis, teres major, deltoid, triceps, and extensor carpi radialis. Movements affected are shoulder adduction and internal rotation, elbow extension, forearm pronation, and wrist flexion. In lower brachial plexus disorders, the muscles affected are abductor pollicis brevis, pectoralis major (sternocostal portion), flexor carpi ulnaris, and first dorsal interosseus. T1 spinal nerve involvement may produce Horner's syndrome, which presents with ptosis of the eyelid and contraction of the pupil on the affected side. Sensory involvement often occurs if the entire brachial plexus is involved (Weber & Lebdusca, 1996). The most common presentation in brachial plexus injuries includes:

- Pain
- Edema
- Limitations in range of motion
- Loss of muscle strength
- Impaired arm and hand functions
- Impaired sensation
- Inability to perform BADLs or IADLs activities
- Limitations affecting work, leisure and social activities performance

Assessment Objectives

The OT will be responsible for assessing occupational performance areas and components. The therapist will be involved in assessment and management of the following areas throughout the course of the patient's acute and rehabilitation phases. All areas assessed will be considered in relation to functional performance to identify realistic client-centered treatment goals.

Assessment of Performance Areas

- Activities of daily living: BADL and IADL skills
- Play and leisure skills
- Work/productivity skills

Assessment of Performance Components

Sensory Processing
- Proprioceptive
- Tactile

Perceptual Processing
- Stereognosis
- Kinesthesia
- Position in space
- Body scheme

Neuromusculoskeletal
- Reflex
- Range of motion
- Muscle tone
- Strength
- Endurance
- Postural control
- Postural alignment

Motor
- Gross coordination
- Bilateral integration
- Motor control
- Praxis
- Fine coordination/dexterity

Cognitive Integration
- Learning
- Generalization

Psychosocial Skills/Psychological Components
- Interests
- Self-concept
- Role performance
- Coping skills

Standardized Assessment Tools

- Pain scales
- Girth measurements or volumetry
- Range of motion test—goniometry
- Manual muscle testing
- Hand function tests—dynamometer and pinch meter could be used

- ADL scales
- Sensory testing
- Work history and job analysis
- Leisure activities checklist

Standardized Tests

- Functional Independence Measure (FIM^{SM})
- Klein-Bell Activities of Daily Living Scale
- Jebson Hand Function Test
- Modified Interest Checklist
- Occupational Performance History Interview
- McGill Pain Questionnaire (MPQ)
- Sensory evaluation form for brachial plexus and hand

Prognosis and Outcome

Prognosis is determined through electrodiagnostic and clinical information. Impairment due to neurapraxia presents the most positive in recovery. In axonotmesis, motor recovery results from axonal sprouting and axon regrowth. Surgical reattachment and the use of nerve jump grafts are indicated in cases of rupture or avulsion.

brain injury See traumatic brain injury.

bulimia nervosa See eating disorders.

burns

Burns are tissue injuries causing protein denaturation, resulting in cell injury or death. The mechanism of injury can be thermal, electrical, chemical, or radioactive agents. The extent of the injury is related to the duration, type, and intensity of action of the agent (Beers & Berkow, 1999).

Etiology

The skin injuries most frequently seen by occupational therapists are burns. All age groups may be seen. The annual incidence of burn-related injuries in the United States is estimated at 1.25 million. Of this number, approximately 50,000 are hospitalized and 5,500 die as a result of their burns (Brigham & McLoughlin, 1996). Just over 50% of the burns reported in a 1988 survey of burn treatment facilities were flame or flash exposure burns; hot liquid or immersion scalds accounted for 35% of the injuries; and electrical contact and chemical burns were approximately 5% of all burn injuries admitted for care.

Symptoms

Superficial partial-thickness: Involves the epidermis and possibly the upper dermis. The burn tissue is characterized by edema, blister formation, acute pain, and erythema.

Deep partial-thickness: Damage to the epidermis and dermis occurs. These burns may leave contractures, hypertrophic scarring, deformity, and dysfunction as they heal.

Full-thickness: Involves loss of the epidermis and all or most of the dermis. These burns do not heal spontaneously, with grafting required for closure in most cases. Development of scarring and hypertrophic scarring results in deformity, limitation in range of motion, and dysfunction.

Severity is measured by the percentage of total body surface area (TBSA) burned. The number of layers of tissue burned measures depth of the burn:

- Small—15% TBSA
- Moderate—15-49% TBSA
- Large—50-69% TBSA
- Massive—More than 70% TBSA

Methods for Calculating the Percentage of Body Burned
Wallace's Rule of Nines (Adult)
  - Head and neck: 9% (4.5% anterior or face, 4.5% posterior)
  - Trunk: anterior 18%, posterior 18%
  - Arms: 9% one (4.5% anterior, 4.5% posterior), 18% both
  - Legs: 18% one (9% anterior, 9% posterior), 36% both
  - Genitalia and perineum: 1%

Stages of Wound Healing
  - Inflammation stage: Lasts 1 to 5 days.
  - Migration and proliferation stage: Begins at 5 days post-injury and lasts up to 14 days.
  - Matrix-forming and remodeling stage: Lasts approximately two months during which time 70% of tensile strength is achieved.

Assessment Objectives

The occupational therapist will be involved in assessment and management of the following performance areas throughout the course of the patient's stay in the acute and rehabilitation setting. All areas assessed will be considered in relation to functional performance. Key areas for assessment include:

- Activities of daily living skills: BADL and IADL
- Work/productivity history, skills, expectations
- Leisure/play skills and interests
- TBSA burned, including type, percentage, location, and depth
- PROM/AROM
- Muscle strength
- Pain tolerance
- Physical endurance, including respiratory status
- Edema
- Transfer and mobility skills
- Ambulation
- Sensory status
- Psychosocial status including: mood, self-concept, coping skills
- Occupational role
- Family values and expectations: cultural values, spiritual support system
- Home environment
- Work environment

Assessment of Performance Areas

- Activities of daily living: Progressive BADL and simple IADL skills
- Work and productive activities: Home management, educational activities, vocational activities, and workplace assessment
- Play or leisure activities

Assessment of Performance Components

Sensoriperceptual Processing

- Tactile
- Proprioceptive
- Visual
- Auditory
- Gustatory

- Olfactory
- Stereognosis
- Kinesthesia
- Pain response
- Body scheme
- Position in space
- Spatial relations
- Topographical orientation

Neuromusculoskeletal
- AROM/PROM
- Muscle tone
- Strength
- Endurance
- Postural control
- Postural alignment
- Soft tissue integrity

Motor
- Gross coordination
- Bilateral integration
- Motor control
- Praxis
- Fine coordination and dexterity
- Visual-motor integration
- Oral-motor control

Cognitive Integration
- Level of arousal
- Orientation
- Recognition
- Attention span
- Spatial operations
- Problem solving
- Learning
- Generalization

Psychosocial Skills
- Values, interests, and self-concept
- Role performance
- Interpersonal skills
- Coping skills

Standardized Assessment Tools

- Barthel Index
- Functional Independence Measure (FIM^{SM})
- Functional Independence Measure for Children (Wee FIM^{SM})
- Modified Interest Checklist
- Pain Apperception Test (PAT)
- Assessment of Motor and Process Skills (AMPS)
- Manual muscle test (MMT) (withheld during acute stages of recovery)
- AROM/PROM test

Prognosis and Outcome

The impact of a burn injury on a person's occupational performance is dependent upon the location, depth, and size of the injury. Maximum level of functional independence is highly correlated with: maximum control of pain facilitating maximization of self-care skills, return to premorbid productive activities (e.g., school, work, and homemaking), and minimization or elimination of deformities.

Reduction and management of hypertrophic scarring to permit performance of self-care routine. Edema control with positioning techniques and/or vascular pressure garments. Return to premorbid roles and occupations.

cancer (neoplasm)

A neoplasm or cancer is a proliferation of abnormal cells in the body. These abnormal cells usually form a solid mass or tumor, as in breast cancer. In leukemia the abnormal cells are lymphocytes, and no mass or tumor develops. The loss of normal control at the cellular level may result in unregulated growth, lack of differentiation, invasion into surrounding tissue, and metastasis to other sites in the body. Cancer (malignancy) can develop in any tissue of any organ at any age (Beers & Berkow, 1999).

Etiology

Cancerous tumors can be divided into two groups: benign or malignant. Benign tumors are composed of normal cells that resemble the host tissue. Usually benign tumors grow slowly, are encapsulated, and do not move to other sites (metastasize). Benign

32

tumors often can be surgically removed, though benign tumors can kill or paralyze if they grow in places where surgery or radiation is not possible or if they compress vital tissue (e.g., tissue in the brain or spinal cord). Malignant tumors are fast-growing cells that are abnormal to the host area. They spread, if left untreated, via the lymphatic and circulatory systems. Cancer tumors can also be classified as low-grade and high-grade tumors. Low-grade tumors tend to grow more slowly than high-grade tumors, and their cellular structures are more uniform and consistent; however, low-grade tumors can be malignant. In contrast, high-grade tumors tend to grow rapidly, tend to metastasize to other organs, and to be resistant to current treatment. Standard treatment interventions for neoplasms or cancer are surgery, radiotherapy, chemotherapy, and transplantation (Reed, 2001).

Symptoms

People of all ages, from infancy through old age, can develop cancers. When people develop cancer, they often lose a significant amount of body weight without intending to. This is because tumors have a higher metabolic rate than normal tissues (Neistadt & Crepeau, 1998). Other sequelae experienced by patients with a diagnosis of cancer are caused by:

- The effect of the primary cancer itself on normal tissues
- The extent and location of the surgery performed to resect or bypass the tumor
- The side effects of the chemotherapy, hormonal therapy, and/or radiation therapy

Assessment Objectives

The occupational therapist will be responsible for assessing occupational performance areas and components. All areas assessed will be considered in relation to functional performance. Key areas for assessment include various performance areas and skills in order to identify realistic client-centered treatment goals.

Assessment of Performance Areas

- Activities of daily living: BADL and IADL skills
- Work and productive activities: home management
- Work or job performance
- Play or leisure activities

Assessment of Performance Components

Perceptual Processing
- Kinesthesia
- Position in space
- Spatial relations
- Topographical orientation
- Stereognosis
- Pain response
- Body scheme
- Spatial relations
- Right-left discrimination
- Visual closure
- Figure ground
- Depth perception

Sensory Processing
- Tactile
- Proprioceptive
- Vestibular
- Auditory

Neuromusculosketetal
- Range of motion
- Muscle tone
- Strength
- Endurance
- Postural alignment
- Postural control
- Soft tissue integrity

Motor
- Gross coordination
- Bilateral integration
- Motor control
- Praxis
- Fine coordination/dexterity
- Laterality
- Visual-motor integration
- Oral-motor control

Cognitive Integration and Cognitive Components (assessment of these components is indicated particularly when there is a neoplasm involving the brain)
- Level of arousal
- Orientation
- Recognition
- Attention span
- Memory
- Sequencing
- Categorization
- Concept formation
- Spatial operations
- Learning
- Generalization

Psychosocial Skills
- Interests
- Self-concept
- Interpersonal skills
- Self-expression
- Coping
- Self-control
- Time management

Standardized Assessment Tools

- Canadian Occupational Performance Measure (COPM), 2nd ed.
- Structured Observational Test of Function (SOTOF)
- Barthel Index
- Assessment of Motor and Process Skills (AMPS)
- Functional Independence Measure (FIM[SM]) version 4.0
- Klein-Bell Activities of Daily Living Scale
- Interests Checklist
- The Chessington O.T. Neurological Assessment Battery (COTNAB)
- The Cognitive Assessment of Minnesota (CAM)
- Lowenstein Occupational Therapy Cognitive Assessment (LOTCA)
- Kohlman Evaluation of Living Skills (KELS)

- Goniometry
- Dynamometer

Other Tests
- Manual Muscle test
- Range of motion test (AROM/PROM)

Prognosis and Outcome

Outcome is dependent on the present clinical status, recent functional history, and response to current functional activity. The person should be able to perform functional and productive tasks, incorporating awareness of energy conservation, work-rest balance, and utilization of assistive and adaptive devices and technology as indicated.

The approach to assessment and management of the patient must be individualized to the person, to the specific disease state, and to the degree of disability. The focus of intervention is prevention, restoration, adaptation, support, or palliation, compensation, and learning/acquisition (Reed, 2001).

cardiac dysfunction, cardiovascular disease

Cardiac dysfunction involves a number of diseases affecting the blood supply, tissues, and muscles in and around the heart (American Heart Association, 1979; Tooth & McKenna, 1996). A number of diseases and symptoms make up cardiac diseases. These include:

- Ischemic heart disease: a condition involving angina, and infarction of myocardial tissue due to arteriosclerotic narrowing of coronary arteries.
- Valvular disease: this occurs when the mitral, tricuspid, and aortic valves fail to function adequately as a result of rheumatic fever or bacterial endocarditis, congestive heart failure, or ischemia.
- Endocarditis: inflammation of heart muscles as a result of valvular diseases, congestive heart failure, and toxic substances in the blood, such as alcohol.
- Cardiac arrest: inadequate ventricular contraction resulting in systematic circulatory failure.
- Pericardial disease: any congenital anomalies and acquired diseases affecting the heart.

Etiology

Causes include thrombus or embolus, arteriosclerosis, bacterial infections that damage the valves, high blood pressure or high fat diet and poor health habits, and high-stress jobs. Myocardial infarction often occurs when a thrombus occludes an artery affected by arthrosclerosis.

Symptoms

Symptoms vary according to the type and severity of the cardiac condition. According to the American Heart Association (1979), cardiac disease can be classified under 4 different severity levels:

Class I: a person has cardiac disease but normal activities do not cause pain or limitations.

Class II: comfortable at rest but experiences pain or slight limitations upon physical activity. The person may experience anginal pain, fatigue, palpitation, or dyspnea upon normal activities.

Class III: cardiac disease leads to marked limitations in the person's physical activities. Comfortable at rest but even less normal activities cause anginal pain, fatigue, palpitation, or dyspnea.

Class IV: these individuals have pain and discomfort even at rest. Very limited in carrying out their daily activities.

Assessment Objectives

The OT will be responsible for assessing occupational performance areas and components. All areas assessed will be considered in relation to functional performance. Key areas for assessment include various performance areas and skills in order to identify realistic client-centered treatment goals.

Assessment of Performance Areas

- Activities of daily living: BADL and simple IADL skills
- Play and leisure skills
- Work/productivity skills

Assessment of Performance Components

Neuromusculoskeletal

- Range of motion
- Muscle tone
- Strength
- Endurance

Motor
- Gross coordination

Cognitive Integration
- Level of arousal
- Orientation
- Attention span
- Memory
- Initiation of activity
- Problem solving
- Sequencing
- Learning
- Generalization

Psychosocial Skills/Psychological Components
- Interests
- Self-concept
- Role performance
- Social conduct
- Interpersonal skills
- Coping skills
- Self-control
- Time management

Standardized Assessment Tools

- ADL scales
- Manual Muscle Test (MMT)
- Range of Motion test (ROM)
- Cognitive evaluation tools
- Occupational performance history
- Work history, job analysis review
- Leisure activities checklist
- Home evaluation for modification and assistive device/equipment recommendation

Standardized Tests
- Assessment of Motor and Process Skills (AMPS)
- Barthel Index
- Beck Depression Inventory
- Canadian Occupational Performance Measure (COPM), 2nd ed.
- Functional Independence Measure (FIM^{SM})

- Kohlman Evaluation of Living Skills (KELS), 3rd ed.
- Modified Interest Checklist
- Occupational Performance History Interview

Prognosis and Outcome

The outcome depends on the severity level of the condition. Early stages of cardiac diseases and conditions can be treated effectively by conditioning exercises and activities, healthy lifestyle training, and prevention of disabilities. In severe stages such as Class III and IV, the prognosis may be that of maintaining function and slowing functional decline.

The primary desired outcome is to improve or maintain ADL independence, muscle strength, endurance, range of motion, ambulation and mobility, and work and leisure skills. Energy conservation techniques may be beneficial. Assistive devices or environmental modifications may be necessary to optimize functional independence. Training family members in appropriate assistance of the client may be necessary.

carpal tunnel syndrome

Carpal tunnel syndrome (CTS) is the result of compression of the median nerve at the wrist, resulting in paresthesis, hyperasthesis, and/or weakness.

Etiology

The carpal tunnel is formed by carpal bones and transverse carpal ligament. Flexor tendons of the hand, fingers, and thumb and median nerve pass through the tunnel. The main cause of CTS is compression of the median nerve in the carpal tunnel between the long flexors and the transverse superficial carpal ligament.

Symptoms

The symptoms manifest as paresthesia or hyperasthesia of the area innervated by the median nerve or atrophy, or weakness of abductor pollicis brevis or opponens pollicis (Burke, Stewart, & Cambre, 1994).

Assessment Objectives

The OT will be responsible for assessing occupational performance areas and components. All areas assessed will be considered in relation to functional performance. Key areas for assessment include various performance areas and skills in order to identify realistic client-centered treatment goals.

Assessment of Performance Areas

- Activities of daily living: BADL and simple IADL skills
- Play and leisure skills
- Work/productivity skills

Assessment of Performance Components

Sensory Processing
- Proprioceptive
- Tactile

Perceptual Processing
- Stereognosis
- Kinesthesia
- Position in space
- Pain response

Neuromusculoskeletal
- Range of motion
- Strength
- Endurance

Motor
- Gross coordination
- Bilateral integration
- Motor control
- Fine coordination/dexterity
- Laterality

Cognitive Integration
- Memory
- Problem solving
- Sequencing
- Learning
- Generalization

Psychosocial Skills/Psychological Components
- Interests
- Role performance
- Coping skills
- Time management

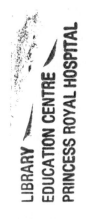

Standardized Assessment Tools

- Goniometer
- Manual muscle test
- Goniometer, dynamometer, pinch meter
- Hand function tests
- Sensory testing
- ADL scales
- Home evaluation
- Assistive devices to evaluate ADL, work, and leisure skills
- Occupational performance history
- Leisure activities checklist

Standardized Tests

- Functional Independence Measure (FIM^SM)
- Barthel Index
- Modified Interest Checklist
- Occupational Performance History Interview
- Jebson Hand Function Test
- Worker Role Inventory
- Self-Esteem Scale
- Purdue Pegboard

Prognosis and Outcome

Prognosis varies depending on the severity of the condition and the amount of joint involvement. Usually the condition improves with rest, splinting, pain medication, activity modifications, and occasionally with surgical decompression.

Hand function, joint range, muscle strength, and daily function can be maintained or increased with medication, exercise, splinting, adaptive equipment, home modifications, and energy conservation techniques.

cerebral palsy

Cerebral palsy is a static disorder with associated sensorimotor impairments; mental retardation; visual, auditory, speech deficits; learning disabilities; and behavioral problems. The type of muscle tone abnormality and the body parts involved often characterize cerebral palsy. The four major types are spastic, athetoid, ataxic, and mixed form. Spastic type occurs in 70% of cases, characterized by the presence of spasticity in specific areas of the body: hemiplegia (one side of the affected), paraplegia/diplegia (both lower extremities are involved), or quadriplegia/tetraplegia (all four extremities are involved). Athetoid type results from basal ganglia involvement and occurs in 20% of the cases. The incidence rate is less than 1:500 live births. The incidence rate has declined in recent years due to improvements in medical technology. Prevalence of mental retardation in all persons with cerebral palsy is estimated to be about 30% (Nelson, 1995).

Etiology

The causes of cerebral palsy could be prenatal, perinatal, or postnatal. Prenatal causes include in utero disorders through exposure to teratogenic drugs or in uterine infections. Perinatal causes include birth trauma, perinatal asphyxia, and neonatal jaundice. Postnatal causes include early childhood disorders such as meningitis, toxins, and head injury. Birth trauma and perinatal asphyxia account for about 15% of the cerebral palsy cases. In terms of the relationship between type and etiology, spastic quadriplegia often results from prenatal causes, and athetoid and ataxic cerebral palsy often result from perinatal causes.

Symptoms

Symptoms vary from minor changes in tone and muscle control, delayed development in motor and/or cognitive skills to severe skeletal deformities limiting all function, lack of postural control, compounded with cognitive and sensory perceptual dysfunction, speech and language disorders, and limitations or lack of social skills and self-help skills. Skills achieved in most cases may not be age appropriate.

Assessment Objectives

The OT will be responsible for assessing the occupational performance areas and relevant components. The assessment should create a baseline to identify realistic client-centered treatment goals.

Assessment of Performance Areas

- Activities of daily living: BADL and simple IADL skills
- Play and leisure skills
- School/educational setting if applicable
- Work/productivity skills

Assessment of Performance Components

Sensory Processing
- Proprioceptive
- Tactile
- Vestibular
- Visual
- Auditory
- Gustatory
- Olfactory

Perceptual Processing
- Kinesthesia
- Position in space
- Body scheme
- Depth perception
- Spatial relations
- Topographical orientation

Neuromusculoskeletal
- Reflex
- Range of motion
- Muscle tone
- Strength
- Endurance
- Postural control
- Postural alignment
- Soft tissue integrity

Motor
- Gross coordination
- Bilateral integration
- Motor control
- Praxis
- Fine coordination/dexterity
- Laterality
- Crossing the midline
- Visual-motor integration
- Oral-motor control

Cognitive Integration
- Level of arousal
- Orientation
- Recognition

- Attention span
- Memory
- Sequencing
- Spatial operations
- Learning
- Generalization

Psychosocial Skills/Psychological Components

- Interests
- Social conduct
- Interpersonal skills
- Self-control

Standardized Assessment Tools

- Developmental scales
- ADL scales
- Sensorimotor scales
- Cognitive and perceptual tests
- Play scales
- Prevocational skills testing

Standardized Tests

- Bayley Scales of Infant Development-II (BSID-II)
- Peabody Developmental Motor Scales (PDMS)
- Functional Independence Measure (FIM^SM) and Functional Independence Measure for Children (WeeFIM^SM)
- Klein-Bell Activities of Daily Living Scale
- Sensory Integration and Praxis Tests (SIPT)
- Developmental Test of Visual Perception, 2nd Edition (DTVP-2)
- Children's Playfulness Scale
- Play Observation
- Vineland Adaptive Behavior Scales-Revised (VABS-R)

Prognosis and Outcome

Evolution of the neuromotor function is possible in the first few years of life. Most children ambulate by the age of 7, rarely later. Persistent primitive reflexes (ATNR, STNR, tonic labyrinthine, Moro's, positive supporting reflex, and extensor posturing) severely affect the development of the milestones of neuromuscular function. Decrease in independence and mobility becomes significant. Abnormal neuromotor control also limits speech and communication skills. Prevention of additional impairments, reduction of disability, and improved social integration of the individual are the main goals of rehabilitation. Total independence may not be achievable for most patients.

cerebrovascular accident, stroke

Cerebrovascular accident (CVA) is an upper motor neuron dysfunction caused by a diminished blood supply to the brain resulting in paralysis of one side of the body (Gillen & Burkhardt, 1998). A lesion in the left cerebral hemisphere (CVA) leads to right hemiplegia and vice versa. Stroke is the third leading cause of death in the United States following heart attack and cancer.

CVA ranges from transient ischemic attacks, which are minor strokes with good recovery of symptoms, to major stroke with residual paralysis.

Etiology

The onset of CVA is sudden. Some of the common factors associated with the incidence of CVA are hypertension, heart disease, cigarette smoking, obesity, heredity, and alcohol consumption. A compromise to the blood supply to the brain, thrombus, embolism, or hemorrhage results in cerebral ischemia and associated physical and cognitive impairments. The most common site of stroke is middle cerebral artery. Other arteries involved include intenal carotid artery, anterior cerebral artery, posterior cerebral artery, cerebellar artery, and vertebrobasilar artery.

Symptoms

Symptoms vary from mild to severe paralysis to the opposite side of the body, sensory dysfunctions, cognitive and perceptual dysfunctions, visual perceptual dysfunctions, and speech and language disorders. These symptoms may be isolated or present in different combinations depending on the severity of the stroke.

Assessment Objectives

The OT will be responsible for assessing occupational performance areas and components. All areas assessed will be considered in relation to functional performance. Key areas for assessment include various performance areas and skills in order to identify realistic client-centered treatment goals.

Assessment of Performance Areas

- Activities of daily living: BADL and simple IADL skills
- Play and leisure skills
- Work/productivity skills

Assessment of Performance Components

Sensory Processing

- Proprioceptive
- Tactile
- Vestibular
- Visual
- Auditory
- Gustatory
- Olfactory

Perceptual Processing

- Stereognosis
- Kinesthesia
- Position in space
- Right-left discrimination
- Form constancy
- Visual closure
- Figure ground
- Body scheme
- Depth perception
- Spatial relations
- Topographical orientation

Neuromusculoskeletal

- Range of motion
- Muscle tone
- Strength
- Endurance
- Postural control
- Postural alignment
- Soft tissue integrity

Motor

- Gross coordination
- Bilateral integration
- Motor control
- Praxis

- Fine coordination/dexterity
- Laterality
- Crossing the midline
- Visual-motor integration
- Oral-motor control

Cognitive Integration

- Level of arousal
- Orientation
- Recognition
- Attention span
- Memory
- Sequencing
- Categorization
- Initiation of activity
- Termination of activity
- Concept formation
- Spatial operations
- Problem solving
- Learning
- Generalization

Psychosocial Skills/Psychological Components

- Values
- Interests
- Self-concept
- Social conduct
- Role performance
- Interpersonal skills
- Self-control
- Self-expression

Standardized Assessment Tools

- ADL scales
- Manual Muscle Test (MMT) (withheld during acute stages of recovery)
- Range of Motion test (ROM)
- Sensory Testing
- Cognitive and perceptual evaluation tools
- Language and communication skills testing
- Occupational performance history
- Work history, job analysis review

- Leisure activities checklist
- Home evaluation for modification and assistive device/equipment recommendation

Standardized Tests
- Assessment of Motor and Process Skills (AMPS)
- Barthel Index
- Brunnstrom Recovery Stages
- Canadian Occupational Performance Measure (COPM), 2nd ed.
- Cognitive Assessment of Minnesota (CAM)
- Functional Independence Measure (FIM[SM])
- Fugl-Meyer Assessment
- Jebson Hand function test
- Kohlman Evaluation of Living Skills (KELS), 3rd ed.
- Loewenstein Occupational Therapy Cognitive Assessment (LOTCA)
- Mini Mental State Evaluation (MMSE)
- Modified Interest Checklist
- Occupational Performance History Interview

Prognosis and Outcome

Recovery takes place for up to 2 years; however, major recovery of function occurs within the first 6 months following the onset.

The primary desired outcome is to improve or maintain ADL independence, muscle strength, endurance, range of motion, ambulation and mobility, and work and leisure skills. Assistive devices or environmental modifications may be necessary to optimize functional independence. Training family members in appropriate assistance of the client may be necessary.

chronic fatigue syndrome

Chronic fatigue syndrome (CFS) is characterized by long-standing, relapsing, severe fatigue without substantial muscle weakness, and without proven psychological or physical causes (Beers & Berkow, 1999).

Etiology

The illness is observed primarily among adults between the ages of 20 and 40 years old. Females demonstrate the symptoms of CFS on a scale of 2:1 to males in the same age ranges. Other names for the syndrome include: chronic Epstein-Barr syndrome, post-viral fatigue syndrome, and chronic fatigue immune dysfunction syndrome. There is controversy about what causes CFS. The illness is thought to be associated with a reaction to viral illness that is complicated by a dysfunctional immune response together with other factors, including gender, age, genetic disposition, prior illness, stress, and environment.

Symptoms

The fatigue impairs daily function and is often exacerbated by exertion, exercise, and other stress. Other symptoms may include: enlarged, painful lymph nodes, sore throat, arthralgia, abdominal and muscle pain, low-grade fever, and difficulty concentrating and sleeping.

Assessment Objectives

The occupational therapist will be responsible for assessing occupational performance areas and components. All areas assessed will be considered in relation to functional performance. Key areas for assessment include various performance areas and skills in order to identify realistic client-centered treatment goals.

Assessment of Performance Areas

• Activities of daily living: BADL and IADL skills
• Work and productive activities: Home management, job performance
• Play or leisure activities

Assessment of Performance Components

Neuromusculoskeletal

• Range of motion
• Strength
• Endurance

Motor

• Gross coordination

Cognitive Integration and Cognitive Components

• Attention span
• Initiation of activity
• Problem solving

Psychosocial Skills

• Interests

- Self-concept
- Interpersonal skills
- Self-expression
- Coping
- Self-control

Standardized Assessment Tools

- Activity Record
- Functional Capacity Evaluation Battery
- Occupational Case Analysis and Interview Rating Scale (OCAIRS)
- Fatigue Severity Scale Human Activity Profile
- Functional Independence Measure v. 4.0 (FIM^{SM})
- Assessment of Motor and Process Skills (AMPS)

Prognosis and Outcome

Outcome is dependent on the present clinical status, recent functional history, and response to current functional activity. The person should be able to perform functional and productive tasks incorporating awareness of energy conservation, work-rest balance, and by utilizing assistive and adaptive devices and technology as indicated.

chronic obstructive pulmonary disorder

Chronic obstructive pulmonary disorder (COPD) is a disease characterized by chronic bronchitis or emphysema and airflow obstruction that is generally progressive, may be accompanied by airway hyperactivity, and may be partially reversible. Asthma is included as a COPD. Clinical symptoms include a chronic or recurrent productive cough and dyspnea. People with COPD tire easily and complain of difficulty talking while involved in functional activities.

Etiology

The causes may include infections, allergens, and skeletal anomalies such as scoliosis, obesity, or disease of the nervous system that affect the muscles that assist breathing. Any factor that contributes to chronic alveolar inflammation, such as smoking, may lead to COPD. Definitive diagnosis is usually made in the 5th or 6th decade of life, though symptoms may be noted earlier.

Symptoms

Chronic bronchitis is characterized by chronic productive cough for at least three months in each of two successive years for which other causes (e.g., infection, cancer, and chronic heart failure) have been ruled out. Emphysema is characterized by abnormal permanent enlargement of the airspaces in the lungs, and asthma is characterized by airway inflammation that is manifested by airway hyper-responsiveness to a variety of stimuli and by airway obstruction that is reversible spontaneously or in response to medical treatment (Beers & Berkow, 1999).

Assessment Objectives

The occupational therapist will be responsible for assessing occupational performance areas and components. All areas assessed will be considered in relation to functional performance. Key areas for assessment include various performance areas and skills in order to identify realistic client-centered treatment goals.

Assessment of Performance Areas

- Activities of daily living: BADL and IADL skills
- Work and productive activities: Home management, care of others, and vocational activities
- Play or Leisure Performance

Assessment of Performance Components

Neuromusculoskeletal

- Range of motion
- Muscle tone
- Strength
- Endurance
- Postural alignment

Psychosocial Skills

- Psychological, social, and self-management

Standardized Assessment Tools

- Borg Scale of Perceived Exertion
- Klein-Bell Activities of Daily Living Scale
- Assessment of Motor and Process Skills (AMPS)
- Functional Independence Measure (FIM^SM)
- Tinetti Test of Balance and Gait
- Berg Balance Test

- Self-Assessment of Leisure Interests
- Interest Checklist
- Self-Esteem Scale
- Tennessee Self-Concept Scale—Revised (TSCS)

Other Tests
  - Range of Motion (AROM/PROM)
  - Manual Muscle Test (MMT)

Prognosis and Outcome

COPD is a chronic disorder that cannot be totally reversed or corrected. Outcome is dependent on the present clinical status, recent functional history, and response to current functional activity.

chronic pain

Pain that persists for extended periods of time (i.e., months or years), that accompanies a disease (e.g., rheumatoid arthritis), or is associated with an injury that has not resolved within an expected time frame is referred to as chronic pain (Turk & Melzack, 1992). Chronic pain complaints can be further differentiated. Chronic, periodic pain is acute but intermittent (e.g., migraine headaches). Chronic, intractable, nonmalignant pain is present most of the time, with intensity varying (e.g., low back pain). Chronic, progressive pain is often associated with malignancies (Turk, Meichenbaum, & Genest, 1983). The most frequently treated types of recurrent painful conditions seen by occupational therapy practitioners include headache, low back pain, arthritis, cancer, and myofacial and extremity pain.

Etiology

Pain has typically been conceptualized as a neurophysiological event that involves a complex pattern of emotional and psychological arousal. Pain has been defined as an unpleasant sensory and emotional experience associated with actual or potential tissue damage or described in terms of such damage (Mersky, 1986).

Symptoms

Effective management of pain relies on a concise, accurate, and multidimensional pain assessment. Overt motor behavior or observable pain responses (e.g., limping), together with well behaviors, are frequently the focus of the evaluation. Persons experiencing pain may rub the pain site, grimace, and/or demonstrate atypical body posturing (Turk, Meichenbaum, & Genest, 1983). Because pain is a private, internal event that cannot be directly observed, assessment of the pain experience is frequently through client self-report of pain intensity, pain affect, and pain location. Pain affect refers to the emotional arousal and disruption caused by the pain experience (Turk & Melzack, 1992). Affective qualities of pain include fear, tension, and autonomic properties, and the reporting of these characteristics may be affected by the client's willingness and/or ability to cooperate and contribute accurate self-reporting. Cultural, familial, and spiritual influences are to be considered by the occupational therapy practitioner in pain assessment and intervention, particularly when the etiology of the pain may be unclear (MacRae & Riley, 1990).

Assessment Objectives

The occupational therapist will be responsible for assessing occupational performance areas and components. All areas assessed will be considered in relation to functional performance. Key areas for assessment include various performance areas and skills in order to identify realistic client-centered treatment goals.

Assessment of Performance Areas

- Activities of daily living: BADL and IADL skills
- Home Management
- Vocational activities: Vocational exploration, job acquisition, and work or job performance
- Play and/or Leisure Activities

Assessment of Performance Components

Sensory Processing
- Tactile
- Proprioceptive

Perceptual Processing
- Pain response
- Body scheme
- Position in space
- Kinesthesia

Neuromusculoskeletal
- Range of motion
- Strength
- Endurance

- Postural control
- Postural alignment

Cognitive Integration
- Attention span
- Initiation of activity
- Memory
- Sequencing

Psychosocial Skills
- Interests
- Self-concept
- Role performance
- Coping skills

Standardized Assessment Tools

- Verbal Rating Scale (VRS)
- Numerical Rating Scale (NRS)
- Visual Analog Scale (VAS)
- McGill Pain Questionnaire (MPQ)
- NPI Interest Checklist
- Occupational Performance History Interview II (OPHI-II)
- Role Checklist, 2nd ed.
- Functional Assessment Screening Questionnaire
- Survey of Pain Attitudes Revised

Prognosis and Outcome

Outcome is dependent on the present clinical status, recent functional history, and response to current functional activity. The person should be able to perform functional and productive tasks incorporating awareness of energy conservation, work-rest balance, and by utilizing assistive and adaptive devices and technology as indicated.

cocaine See prenatal exposure to cocaine.

coma

Coma is a state in which a person is unarousable and any response to repeated stimuli is only a primitive avoidance reflex. In profound coma, all brainstem and myotatic reflexes may be absent (Beers & Berkow, 1999).

Etiology

Since impaired consciousness is but one manifestation of an underlying disease or injury, its mode of onset, duration, intensity, and other characteristics depend on the cause. Possible causes are many and varied but depend ultimately on diffuse suppression of neuronal function or damage to structures in the brainstem, directly or secondarily to increased intracranial pressure. Some of the most common causes are cranial trauma, stroke, poisoning (particularly by carbon monoxide or barbiturates), epilepsy, and diabetic acidosis. Other causes include cerebral hypoxia (secondary to heart failure, severe anemia, heart block), hypoglycemic and other forms of shock, infections (particularly meningeal and pulmonary), and expanding brain lesions.

Symptoms

Assessment should start while the patient is in the intensive care unit (ICU), and should be closely coordinated with the physician, nursing staff, and the physical therapy staff. It is important for the therapist to be aware of the potential medical and surgical management problems and precautions before beginning the evaluation. Blood pressure, pulse rate, and oxygen saturation rate should be closely monitored, and the assessment should be withheld if they are not within the parameters established by the attending physician. Those patients with an increase in intracranial pressure (ICP) must be watched closely. The occupational therapy evaluation must stop if the ICP rises above the criteria established by the attending physician. It is important to observe the patient after the assessment session to identify any delayed ICP responses. Clinical observations such as changes in neurological status (including papillary changes), diaphoresis (excessive sweating), vomiting, behavioral changes, changes in posture, and changes in respiratory patterns should continually be made as the occupational therapy assessment is progressing.

Assessment Objectives

It is essential to understand how severity of injury is assessed because management of the coma patient varies significantly depending upon the severity of the injury to the brain. There continues to be no absolute measure of severity of brain injury, though duration and depth of coma, and length of post-traumatic amnesia (PTA) are accepted criteria. The method most used by professionals to categorize the levels of consciousness in the acute phases of recovery following trauma to the brain is the Glasgow Coma Scale (Jennett & Teasdale, 1981). As the patient stabilizes and improves, the OT may use the Rancho Los Amigos Scale of Cognitive Functioning (1980), a behavioral rating system that assesses cognitive recovery. The occupational therapist will be responsible for assessing occupational performance areas and components. All areas assessed will be considered in relation to functional performance. Key areas for assessment include various performance areas and skills in order to identify realistic client-centered treatment goals.

Assessment of Performance Areas

- Activities of daily living: BADL and IADL skills appropriate for specific level of recovery
- Work and productive activities: Home management and vocational activities
- Play or leisure activities

Assessment of Performance Components

Sensory Processing
- Tactile
- Proprioceptive
- Vestibular
- Visual
- Auditory
- Gustatory
- Olfactory

Perceptual Processing
- Stereognosis
- Kinesthesia
- Pain response
- Body scheme
- Right-left discrimination
- Position in space
- Figure ground
- Depth perception
- Spatial relations
- Topographical orientation

Neuromusculoskeletal
- Reflex
- Range of motion
- Muscle tone
- Strength
- Endurance
- Postural control
- Postural alignment
- Soft tissue integrity

Motor
- Gross coordination
- Bilateral integration
- Motor control
- Praxis
- Visual-motor integration
- Oral-motor control

Cognitive Integration
- Level of arousal
- Orientation
- Recognition
- Attention span
- Initiation of activity
- Termination of activity
- Memory and sequencing
- Categorization
- Concept formation
- Spatial operations
- Problem solving
- Learning
- Generalization

Psychosocial Skills
- Interests
- Social conduct
- Interpersonal skills
- Self-control

Standardized Assessment Tools

- Glasgow Coma Scale (GCS)
- Innsbruck Coma Scale (ICS)

- Rancho Los Amigos Cognitive Functioning Scale
- Functional Independence Measure (FIM^{SM})
- Assessment of Motor and Process Skills (AMPS)
- Barthel Index
- Katz Index of ADL
- Klein-Bell Activities of Daily Living Scale
- Berg Balance Test
- Tinetti Balance Test
- Coma/Near Coma Scale (CNC)
- Coma Recovery Scale (CRS)
- Sensory Stimulation Assessment Measure (SSAM)
- Western Sensory Stimulation Profile (WNSSP)
- The Cognitive Assessment of Minnesota (CAM)
- Lowenstein Occupational Therapy Cognitive Assessment (LOTCA)

Other Tools
  - Goniometry
  - Dynamometer
  - Pinch meter
  - Range of Motion (AROM/PROM)
  - Manual Muscle test (MMT)

Prognosis and Outcome

Due to the uncertainty accompanying brain injury, it is difficult to predict a level of recovery. The recovery from brain injury and coma happens in stages. The first stage includes intensive, lifesaving medical and technical procedures that occur in an acute care facility immediately following the trauma or cerebral insult. After the acute care stage, the challenge of recovery then shifts to focus on the remaining stages of physical, occupational, and neuropsychological restoration. The rate of recovery is most rapid during the initial weeks of the brain injury or after the person awakens from the coma. It is important that the period of rapid recovery does not mislead both the family and treatment staff to predict continued recovery. Unfortunately, when there is a slowdown of recovery after this stage, it can be very difficult for families. It is essential to note that each individual progresses at his or her own rate of recovery. It is important to note that a slowdown in progress does not mean an end to recovery. Continued gains in function have been reported even several years after the injury. There are many factors that will affect the level of recovery after brain injury, such as: age at time of incident, severity and the part of the brain affected by the injury, length of time in coma, preexisting personality characteristics, quality of prehospital (paramedic/EMS) and hospital care, speed of entry into brain injury rehabilitation program, the nature of the support network, and involvement of family.

deconditioned/generalized debility, weakness

Deconditioning is a common problem that can delay, interrupt, or undermine an individual's ability to participate in rehabilitation (Bachelder, 1994). Debility can be defined as multiple changes in organ systems resulting in the depletion of organ reserves (Seibens, 1990). The degree and complexity of the functional consequences of deconditioning are due at least in part to each of the following components:

- Age-related changes
- Premorbid levels of activity
- Chronic, concurrent medical conditions
- Lengthy bed rest

The debilitating pattern of inactivity and disuse occur earlier and with greater severity in older adults (Seibens, 1990). Deconditioning may go unnoticed during the acute stage of recovery from an illness or injury, since most patients do not place significant stress on their cardiopulmonary or muscular system (Brummel-Smith, 1990).

Etiology

Limitations in endurance may interfere significantly with an individual's ability to participate in all of the tasks that define his or her roles. A newly acquired disability typically has an impact on endurance, even in the absence of cardiopulmonary complications. A limitation in strength, sensation, muscle tone, range of motion, or a visual-spatial impairment can require the client to expend more energy for the completion of self-care tasks than was required prior to the disability or onset of the condition. Many older adults tend to lead more sedentary lifestyles than their younger counterparts, which may also contribute to declines in cardiovascular fitness (Lewis & Bottomley, 1996). As a result, the elder may have little, if any, reserve available for the extra demands of a newly acquired disability or condition.

Symptoms

Deconditioning may manifest in the older adult patient in one or all of the following signs and symptoms:

- Exaggerated heart rate
- Significant changes in blood pressure from resting rate
- Decreased muscle power
- Decreased physical endurance
- Reduced ability to participate in self-care activities
- Fatigue
- Diminished motivation for engagement and activity

Assessment Objectives

The occupational therapist will be responsible for assessing occupational performance areas and components. All areas assessed will be considered in relation to functional performance. Key areas for assessment include various performance areas and skills in order to identify realistic client-centered treatment goals.

Assessment of Performance Areas

- Activities of daily living: BADL and IADL skills
- Home Management
- Work productivity: prevocational and vocational skills
- Leisure Activities

Assessment of Performance Components

Sensory Processing

- Tactile
- Proprioceptive
- Vestibular
- Visual
- Auditory

Perceptual Processing

- Stereognosis
- Kinesthesia
- Pain response
- Position in space
- Depth perception

- Spatial relations
- Topographical orientation

Neuromusculoskeletal
- Range of motion (passive and active) for all joints
- Muscle tone
- Strength
- Endurance
- Postural control
- Postural alignment
- Soft tissue integrity

Motor
- Gross coordination
- Laterality
- Bilateral integration
- Motor control
- Praxis
- Fine coordination/dexterity
- Oral-motor control (swallow)

Cognitive Integration
- Level of arousal
- Orientation
- Recognition
- Attention span
- Initiation of activity
- Memory
- Sequencing
- Spatial operations
- Problem solving
- Learning

Psychosocial Skills
- Interests
- Self-concept
- Role performance
- Self-expression
- Coping skills

Standardized Assessment Tools

- Activity Record
- Functional Capacity Evaluation Battery

- Occupational Case Analysis and Interview Rating Scale (OCAIRS)
- Fatigue Severity Scale
- Human Activity Profile
- Functional Independence Measure v. 4.0 (FIM^{SM})
- Manual Muscle Test (MMT)
- Range of Motion test (AROM and PROM)
- Klein-Bell ADL Scale
- Berg Balance Test
- Tinetti Test of Balance and Gait
- Rhomberg Test of Balance
- Sensory Testing
- Self-Esteem Scale
- Assessment of Motor and Process Skills (AMPS)
- Canadian Occupational Performance Measure (COPM)

Prognosis and Outcome

When endurance and deconditioning limit the person's ability to participate fully in tasks that the person finds meaningful, assessment should lead to treatment. Treatment should begin with a graded program to increase endurance by progressively increasing the number and duration of activities successfully completed in a treatment session or treatment day. Once this goal has been reached, an endurance program to enhance general conditioning is indicated to improve the endurance threshold to a level above that which is required by the individual to complete his or her daily occupations without feeling exhausted. This graded approach to exercise and self-care activities will also serve to provide some reserves in the event that the person sustains another disability or deconditioning event (Dean & Ross, 1994).

dementia (non-Alzheimer's type)

Dementia is a structurally caused permanent or progressive decline in intellectual function that interferes significantly with the person's normal social and functional activity. The essential feature of a dementia is the development of multiple cognitive deficits that include memory impairment together with at least one of the following cognitive disturbances: aphasia, apraxia, agnosia, or a disturbance in executive functioning (American Psychiatric Association, 1994).

Listed in the *DSM-IV* are 11 types of dementia (American Psychiatric Association, 1994). Alzheimer's disease is covered under its own heading in this text. Other dementias include vascular dementia (multi-infarct dementia) and dementia secondary to:

- Head injury
- HIV
- Parkinson's disease
- Vascular disease (multi-infarct)
- Huntington's disease
- Pick's disease
- Creutzfeldt-Jakob disease
- Substance abuse
- Multiple etiologies

Etiology

Static dementia is generally caused by one major event of catastrophic proportions, such as stroke, myocardial infarction with cardiac arrest, or traumatic head injury. Progressive dementias are classified into three primary categories (examples of each are not all inclusive):

1. Metabolic or Toxic
- Anoxia
- Vitamin B12 deficiency
- Chronic drug or alcohol abuse
- Hypothyroidism
- Liver and/or lung failure

2. Structural
- Alzheimer's disease
- Amyotrophic lateral sclerosis
- Brain trauma or tumor
- Multiple sclerosis
- Multi-infarct dementia
- Parkinson's disease
- Dementia with Lewy bodies
- Normal-pressure hydrocephalus

3. Infectious
- Bacterial endocarditis
- Creutzfeldt-Jakob disease
- HIV-related disorders

- Neurosyphilis
- Tuberculosis
- Viral encephalitis

Symptoms

Dementia with Lewy bodies is considered the second most frequent cause of dementia in elderly adults. A neurodegenerative disorder, Lewy body dementia is associated with abnormal structures (Lewy bodies) found in certain areas of the brain. Symptoms can range from traditional Parkinsonian effects, such as loss of spontaneous movement (bradykinesia), rigidity, tremor, and shuffling gait, to effects similar to those of Alzheimer's disease, such as acute confusion, memory loss, and loss or fluctuation of cognition. Visual hallucinations may be one of the first symptoms noted, and patient may suffer from other psychiatric disturbances such as delusions and depression. Onset of the disorder usually occurs in older adults, though younger people can be affected as well. *Multi-infarct dementia* (MID), a common cause of dementia in the elderly, occurs when blood clots block small blood vessels in the brain and destroy brain tissue. This disease can cause stroke, dementia, migraine-like headaches, and psychiatric disturbances. Symptoms of MID, which often develop in a graduated progression, include confusion, problems with recent memory, wandering or getting lost in familiar places, loss of bladder or bowel control, and emotional problems including lability, difficulty following instructions, and money management. Usually the damage is so slight that the change is noticeable only as a series of small steps or incidents. MID, which typically begins between the ages of 60 and 75, affects men more often than women (National Institute on Aging, 1995). *Creutzfeldt-Jakob disease* (CJD) is a rare, degenerative, and ultimately fatal brain disorder. It affects about one person in every one million people per year worldwide; in the United States there are about 200 cases per year. CJD usually appears in later life and runs a rapid course. Typically, onset of symptoms occurs about age 60, and about 90% of patients die within one year. In the early stages of the disease, patients may have failing memory, behavioral changes, lack of coordination, and visual disturbances. As the disease progresses, mental deterioration becomes pronounced and involuntary movements, blindness, weakness of extremities, and coma may occur (National CJD Surveillance Unit, 2001).

Assessment Objectives

The occupational therapist will be responsible for assessing occupational performance areas and components. All areas assessed will be considered in relation to functional performance. Key areas for assessment include various performance areas and skills in order to identify realistic client-centered treatment goals.

Assessment of Performance Areas

- Activities of daily living: BADL and simple IADL skills
- Home management
- Leisure

Assessment of Performance Components

Sensory Processing

- Tactile
- Proprioceptive
- Vestibular
- Visual
- Auditory
- Olfactory

Perceptual Processing

- Stereognosis
- Kinesthesia
- Pain response
- Body scheme
- Right-left discrimination
- Form constancy
- Position in space
- Visual closure
- Figure ground
- Depth perception
- Spatial relations
- Topographical orientation

Neuromusculoskeletal

- Range of motion
- Muscle tone
- Strength
- Endurance
- Postural control

- Postural alignment
- Soft tissue integrity

Motor
- Gross coordination
- Crossing the midline
- Laterality
- Bilateral integration
- Motor control
- Praxis
- Fine coordination/dexterity
- Visual-motor integration
- Oral-motor control

Cognitive Integration and Cognitive Components
- Level of arousal
- Orientation
- Recognition
- Attention span
- Initiation of activity
- Termination of activity
- Memory and sequencing
- Spatial operations
- Problem solving
- Learning
- Generalization

Psychosocial Skills
- Interests
- Social conduct
- Interpersonal skills
- Self-expression
- Coping
- Self-control
- Role performance

Standardized Assessment Tools

- Mini Mental State Exam (MMSE)
- Middlesex Elderly Assessment of Mental State (MEAMS)
- The Cognitive Assessment of Minnesota (CAM)
- Kohlman Evaluation of Living Skills (KELS)
- Allen Cognitive Level Scale (ACLS)
- Assessment of Motor and Process Skills (AMPS)

- Functional Independence Measure (FIM^{SM})
- Berg Balance Test
- Tinetti Test of Balance and Gait
- Rhomberg Test of Balance
- Sensory Testing
- Self-Esteem Scale
- Geriatric Depression Scale
- Self-Assessment of Leisure Interests
- Occupational Therapy Home Evaluation

Prognosis and Outcome

The prognosis is not good. The client's functional and cognitive course is usually in steady decline. Dementia is considered a progressive and ultimately terminal disease process. The length of the course is variable. Formal and informal caregiver support systems can combine successfully to assist the client and his or her family to adapt and learn compensatory strategies for dealing with the loss of cognitive skills. It is valuable to understand that dementia is not one condition; rather it is a variable set of conditions that can be exhibited in complex and changing sets of symptoms. There is no one customary or typical pattern of problems or issues that are displayed by the person with dementia. Because of the many and varied causes of dementia, one might anticipate a wide variety of presenting symptoms. Family members and caregivers can benefit from support groups, counseling, and respite services.

depression

Depression is an affective disorder characterized by mood disturbance, psychomotor dysfunction, and vegetative symptoms (American Psychiatric Association, 1994). Depression can be unipolar (depressive) or part of bipolar (manic-depressive) disorder.

Etiology

A number of theories exist about the causes of depression. According to psychoanalytical theories, depression occurs due to the loss of a loved one or an object. According to behavioral theories depression occurs as a result of a negative person-environment interaction and negative cognitive patterns of thinking. Biochemical theories view depression as a result of decreased neurotransmitters at the synoptic junction. Sociological theories describe depression as a result of stresses associated with life roles and a person's inability to cope with demands associated with life roles. Existential theories view depression as a result of one's inability to find meaning in life. It is estimated that about 25% of the population experiences depression at some point in life and women are affected more frequently than men.

Symptoms

Symptoms include:

- Lack of interest in daily activities
- Loss of appetite and weight loss
- Sleep disorders or insomnia
- Inability to perform work-related tasks
- Loss of interest in leisure activities
- Psychomotor retardation
- Agitation or restlessness
- Lack of physical endurance
- Visual or auditory hallucinations
- Difficulty initiating or attending to tasks
- Recurrent thoughts about death and suicide
- Difficulty with decision making and problem solving
- Poor self-concept and lack of self-confidence
- Feelings of helplessness and hopelessness
- Social withdrawal
- Feelings of guilt and worthlessness
- Frequent crying
- Inability to express emotions of feelings
- Dependence with otherwise routine daily tasks

Assessment Objectives

The OT will be responsible for assessing occupational performance areas and components. All areas assessed will be considered in relation to functional performance. Key areas for assessment include various performance areas and skills in order to identify realistic client-centered treatment goals.

Assessment of Performance Areas

- Activities of daily living: BADL and simple IADL skills
- Play and leisure skills
- Work/productivity skills

Assessment of Performance Components

The following performance components and skills should be assessed in order to identify realistic client-centered treatment goals:

• Activities of daily living
• Work history and skills
• Leisure skills and interests
• Physical fitness and endurance
• Gross and fine motor skills
• Attention and concentration span
• Problem solving and memory
• Decision making and organization skills
• Mood and affect
• Communications skills
• Social roles and skills
• Self-concept and values
• Perceptual skills

Standardized Assessment Tools

• ADL scales
• Occupational performance history
• Work history, job analysis review
• Leisure activities checklist
• Cognitive scales
• Perception evaluation scales

Standardized Tests

• Assessment of Motor and Process Skills (AMPS), 2nd ed.
• Mini Mental State Examination (MMSE)
• Modified Interest Checklist
• Occupational Performance History Interview
• Self-Esteem Scale
• Worker Role Inventory
• Allen Cognitive Level Test
• Canadian Occupational Performance Measure (COPM)
• Kohlman Evaluation of Living Skills (KELS) (3rd ed.)
• Beck Depression Inventory
• Burns Depression Checklist
• Internal-External Locus of Control Scale
• Social Readjustment Rating Scale

Prognosis and Outcome

A person may be able to regain independence in daily function and occupational roles with psychotropic medication and functional skills training.

developmental disabilities—adults

According to the Mental Retardation Facilities and Community Health Centers Construction Act (1963) and the Developmental Disabilities Assistance and Bill of Rights Amendments of 1987, individuals with developmental disabilities present with severe physical or mental disabilities. There may also be a combination of physical and mental impairments. To be classified as a developmental disability, it should occur before the age of 22 and must present indefinitely. The results of the disability should be evident in daily life activities such as self-care, communication, mobility, learning, independent living skills, and economic independence. Many adults with developmental disabilities present with autism, mental retardation, neurological impairments, epilepsy, and other lifelong sensory-motor disabilities.

Etiology

The cause of developmental disability varies. Some of the common causes leading to developmental disability include:

- Birth trauma
- In utero growth retardation
- Infectious diseases
- Accidents
- Substance abuse and addictions by the mother leading to defective fetal development
- Genetic disorders

Symptoms

Delay of normal developmental milestones; if present with learning problems it will lead to difficulty transferring learning from lower skills to more advanced skills.

ADL, Communication, and Leisure

The individual may not have mastered the learning of self-care tasks leading to inadequate self-care skills, poor grooming and hygiene skills, inability to live independently in the community, and inadequate homemaking skills. Most of these individuals will require some form of assistance or supervision for performing their daily self-care and community living tasks.

Language

- Slow development of speech
- Difficulty learning new vocabulary or naming familiar items
- Uses two- or three-word phrases instead of strings of words
- Speech is difficult to understand
- Difficulty expressing wants or needs
- Trouble following even simple directions
- Undeveloped work skills and employment skills, and display poor or nonexistent work habits and skills
- Inadequate leisure skills or may not have developed any leisure skills

Sensorimotor

- The person may have gross and fine motor deficits, low muscle tone, decreased eye-hand coordination and dexterity. May have sensory integration dysfunction such as reflex integration and vestibular, tactile, and proprioceptive and visual deficits.
- Difficulty manipulating small objects (using pencil/crayon); poor balance; awkwardness with jumping, running, or climbing; poor sense of personal space.
- The person may have stereotypic behaviors such as rocking, face or eye rubbing, and/or finger flicking, as a result of poor integration of vestibular, tactile, and proprioceptive input.

Cognitive

- Inability to learn from incidental experience. Requires structured situations for learning tasks. May have mental retardation and associated cognitive disabilities. May exhibit poor eye contact and poor attention span. May not have task-oriented and goal-directed behaviors. Difficulty understanding cause and effect; problems with sequencing and one-to-one correspondence; difficulty with basic concepts (e.g., size, shape, and color). Easily distracted, acts impulsively, displays poor organizational skills.

Psychosocial

- Poor learning skills and imitation skills. May have poor impulse control and poor self-perception. May exhibit lack of social development to appropriate age level and lack of social play skills. May exhibit unacceptable behaviors such as pushing, throwing things, hitting self/others, or self-injurious behaviors

- Poor stress handling skills and coping skills; inability to handle self in social situations and may withdraw self from social situations
- Exhibit difficulty in relating to authority and difficulty relating to peers
- Inability to manage time without assistance
- Difficulty with (or disinterest in) peer socialization; overly aggressive or withdrawn; sudden and extreme mood changes; frequent crying or tantrums; poor frustration tolerance

Assessment Objectives

The OT will be responsible for assessing occupational performance areas and components that affect independence in areas of personal, social, prevocational, and vocational pursuits. All areas assessed will be considered in relation to functional performance. Key areas for assessment include various performance areas and skills in order to identify realistic client-centered treatment goals.

Assessment of Performance Areas

- Activities of daily living: BADL and simple IADL skills
- Leisure/play skills
- School/educational setting if applicable
- Work/productivity skills

Assessment of Performance Components

Sensory Processing

- Proprioceptive
- Tactile
- Vestibular
- Visual
- Auditory
- Gustatory
- Olfactory

Perceptual Processing

- Stereognosis
- Kinesthesia
- Position in space

- Right-left discrimination
- Figure ground
- Body scheme
- Depth perception
- Spatial relations
- Topographical orientation

Neuromusculoskeletal
- Range of motion
- Muscle tone
- Strength
- Endurance
- Postural control

Motor
- Gross coordination
- Bilateral integration
- Motor control
- Praxis
- Fine coordination/dexterity
- Laterality
- Visual-motor integration
- Oral-motor control

Cognitive Integration
- Level of arousal
- Orientation
- Recognition
- Attention span
- Memory
- Sequencing
- Categorization
- Initiation of activity
- Termination of activity
- Spatial operations
- Problem solving
- Learning
- Generalization

Psychosocial Skills/Psychological Components
- Interests
- Social conduct
- Interpersonal skills

- Self-control
- Self-expression

Standardized Assessment Tools

- ADL scales
- Developmental scales
- Hand function tests
- Leisure scales
- Cognitive and perceptual tests
- Sensory integration tests
- Prevocational/vocational evaluation

Standardized Tests

- Adult Skills Evaluation Survey for Persons with Mental Retardation (ASES)
- Assessment of Motor and Process Skills (AMPS)
- Developmental Test of Visual Perception, 2nd Edition (DTVP-2)
- Peabody Developmental Motor Scales (PDMS)
- Functional Independence Measure (FIM[SM])
- Crawford Small Parts Dexterity Test (1981 Revised)
- Sensory Integration and Inventory—Revised for Individuals with Developmental Disabilities
- Vineland Adaptive Behavior Scales-Revised (VABS-R)

Prognosis and Outcome

The prognosis of adults with developmental disabilities may vary depending on their level of disabilities. Building on the person's abilities and strengths and teaching simple self-care and community living skills can lead to increased independence in ADL and IADL tasks. Speech and language programs and psychological services also may be incorporated as needed in order to improve one's communication and psychosocial skills. Simple vocational and prevocational skills can be taught in order to perform vocational and prevocational tasks. Teach leisure skills and interests. A person can learn socially acceptable behaviors, including basic conversation skills and cooperative behavior.

diabetes mellitus

Diabetes mellitus is a syndrome characterized by hyperglycemia resulting from absolute or relative impairment in insulin secretion and/or insulin reaction (Beers & Berkow, 1999). Chronic hyperglycemia causes damage to the eyes, kidneys, nerves, heart, and blood vessels. The etiology and pathophysiology leading to the hyperglycemia, however, are markedly different among patients with diabetes mellitus, dictating different prevention strategies, diagnostic screening methods, and treatments.

Over 95% of persons with type 1 diabetes mellitus develop the disease before the age of 25, with an equal incidence in both sexes and an increased prevalence in the white population.

Type 2 diabetes mellitus is the most common form and is highly associated with a family history of diabetes, older age, obesity, and lack of exercise. It is more common in women, especially women with a history of gestational diabetes, and in blacks, Hispanics, and Native Americans.

Types of diabetes mellitus of various known etiologies are grouped together under "other specific types."

Etiology

Type 1 diabetes mellitus (formerly called type I, IDDM, or juvenile diabetes) is characterized by beta cell destruction caused by an autoimmune process, usually leading to absolute insulin deficiency. A family history of type 1 diabetes mellitus, gluten enteropathy (celiac disease), or other endocrine disease is often found.

Type 2 diabetes mellitus (formerly called NIDDM, type II, or adult-onset) is characterized by insulin resistance in peripheral tissue and an insulin secretory defect of the beta cell. Insulin resistance and hyperinsulinemia eventually lead to impaired glucose tolerance. Defective beta cells become exhausted, further fueling the cycle of glucose intolerance and hyperglycemia. The etiology of type 2 diabetes mellitus is multifactorial and probably genetically based, but it also has strong behavioral components (Mayfield, 1998).

Symptoms

- General weakness and loss of weight
- Specific muscle weakness and atrophy
- Limited range of motion
- Sensory loss of touch, temperature, pain
- Complaints of paresthesias, hyperesthesia

- Loss of vision and other eye changes
- Cognitive deficits from secondary medical diagnoses

Assessment Objectives

The OT will be responsible for assessing occupational perform-ance areas and components. All areas assessed will be considered in relation to functional performance. Key areas for assessment include various performance areas and skills in order to identify realistic client-centered treatment goals.

Assessment of Performance Areas

- Activities of daily living: BADL and simple IADL skills
- Play and leisure skills
- School/educational setting if applicable
- Work/productivity skills

Assessment of Performance Components

Sensory Processing

- Proprioceptive
- Tactile
- Visual

Perceptual Processing

- Stereognosis
- Depth perception

Neuromusculoskeletal

- Strength
- Endurance
- Soft tissue integrity

Motor

- Fine coordination/dexterity

Cognitive Integration

- Problem solving
- Learning
- Generalization

Psychosocial Skills/Psychological Components

- Interests
- Role performance

Standardized Assessment Tools

- Manual Muscle Test (MMT)
- Range of Motion test (ROM)

- Sensory Testing
- ADL scales
- Home Evaluation for modification and assistive device/equipment recommendation
- Occupational performance history
- Work history, job analysis review
- Leisure activities checklist

Standardized Tests
- Functional Independence Measure (FIM^{SM})
- Barthel Index
- Modified Interest Checklist
- Occupational Performance History Interview
- Jebson Hand Function Test

Prognosis and Outcome

Complications are associated with poorly controlled diabetes in most cases and include retinopathy, peripheral neuropathy, and nephropathy. Ulcers on the feet, which in severe cases can develop into gangrene, are another major risk. Cardiovascular symptoms can include orthostatic intolerance or cardiac arrhythmias (Buschbacher, 1996). Atherosclerosis, hypertension and other cardiovascular disorders, and cataracts are other associated risk factors in diabetics. Early diagnosis and treatment can significantly improve the patient's quality of life. Social awareness and education of symptoms and management are key to reducing the incidence and severity of complications.

Down syndrome

Down syndrome, also known as trisomy 21, trisomy G, or mongolism, is a chromosomal disorder resulting in mental retardation, a characteristic facies, and other features such as microcephaly (small head), and short stature. There are three types of Down syndrome: trisomy, translocation, and mosaicism. The name trisomy 21 is derived because an extra twenty-first chromosome, or the translocation of part of the twenty-first chromosome onto another chromosome, usually causes the condition. Down syndrome is the most common type of chromosomal abnormality occurring in the autosomes, and is responsible for about one-third of all cases of moderate-to-severe mental retardation.

Down syndrome

Etiology

About 1 in every 700 babies born alive has Down syndrome (Hayes & Batshaw, 1993). The risk is greatest with older parents: the chances rise from 1 such birth in 2,000 among 25-year-old mothers to 1 in 40 for women over 45. The risk also rises with the father's age, especially with men over 50. The exact cause of Down syndrome is not completely understood. DNA analysis has demonstrated that the extra chromosome seems to come from the mother's ovum in 95% of the cases (Antonarakis & Down Syndrome Collaborative Group, 1991); the other 5% of the cases seem to be related to the father.

Symptoms

The most obvious physical characteristic associated with the disorder is a downward-sloping skinfold at the inner corners of the eyes. Other signs are a small head (microcephaly), a flat nose, a protruding tongue, motor retardation, and defective heart, gastrointestinal tract, eyes, and ears.

Assessment Objectives

The occupational therapist will be responsible for assessing occupational performance areas and components. All areas assessed will be considered in relation to functional performance. Key areas for assessment include various performance areas and skills in order to identify realistic client-centered treatment goals.

Assessment of Performance Areas

- Activities of daily living: BADL skills
- Educational activities
- Prevocational activities
- Play or Leisure activities

Assessment of Performance Components

Sensorimotor
- Sensory and perceptual processing

Neuromusculoskeletal
- Reflex
- ROM
- Muscle tone
- Strength
- Endurance

- Postural control
- Postural alignment

Motor

- Gross coordination
- Crossing the midline
- Laterality, bilateral integration
- Motor control
- Praxis
- Fine coordination and dexterity
- Visual-motor integration
- Oral-motor control

Cognitive Integration

- Recognition
- Attention span
- Memory and sequencing
- Spatial operations
- Problem solving
- Learning
- Generalization

Psychosocial Skills

- Interests
- Self-expression

Self-Management

- Coping skills
- Self-control

Standardized Assessment Tools

- Erhardt Developmental Prehension Assessment-Revised
- Bayley Scales of Infant Development-II (BSID-II)
- Bruininks-Oseretsky Test of Motor Proficiency (BOTMP)
- Gesell Developmental Schedules—Revised
- Peabody Developmental Motor Scales
- Range of Motion test (AROM/PROM)
- Manual Muscle Test (MMT)

Prognosis and Outcome

The prognosis for children with Down syndrome is brighter than
was once thought. Many live at home until adulthood and then
enter small group homes or adult foster homes. Many can support
themselves; they tend to do well in structured job situations. More

than 70% of people with Down syndrome live into their sixties, but they are at special risk of developing Alzheimer's disease (Hayes & Batshaw, 1993).

Duchenne's muscular dystrophy

Muscular dystrophy is an inherited progressive muscle disorder, which is characterized by muscle weakness. Duchenne's muscular dystrophy (DMD) is a type of muscular dystrophy that is inherited and is characterized by destruction of muscle fibers that are replaced by connective tissue (Tomchek, 1999). There are different types of muscular dystrophy such as Duchenne's, fascioscapulohumeral, limb-girdle, and Becker's muscular dystrophy.

Etiology

DMD is an inherited disorder that affects only males, and the mother carries the defective X gene.

Symptoms

The symptoms include frequent falls, difficulty standing up and climbing stairs, difficulty running, difficulty getting up to standing position, a waddling gait, toe walking, and lordosis. A person might get to standing by climbing through the support of his legs (Gower's sign). Symptoms start in boys anywhere between 3 and 7 years of age. Loss of self-care skills and functional independence results from muscle weakness.

Assessment Objectives

The OT will be responsible for assessing occupational perform-ance areas and components. All areas assessed will be considered in relation to functional performance. Key areas for assessment include various performance areas and skills in order to identify realistic client-centered treatment goals.

Assessment of Performance Areas

- Activities of daily living: BADL and simple IADL skills
- Play and leisure skills
- Work/productivity skills

Assessment of Performance Components

Sensory Processing
- Proprioceptive

Neuromusculoskeletal
- Reflex
- Range of motion
- Muscle tone
- Strength
- Endurance
- Postural control
- Postural alignment
- Soft tissue integrity

Motor
- Gross coordination
- Bilateral integration
- Motor control
- Fine coordination/dexterity

Cognitive Integration
- Attention span
- Spatial operations
- Problem solving
- Learning
- Generalization

Psychosocial Skills/Psychological Components
- Values
- Interests
- Self-concept
- Role performance
- Social conduct
- Interpersonal skills
- Self-expression
- Coping skills
- Time management
- Self-control

Standardized Assessment Tools
- ADL scales
- Occupational performance history
- School functional assessment
- Leisure activities checklist
- Muscle Test (goniometer, pinch meter, dynamometer, hand function tests)
- Range of Motion test (ROM)

- Sensory Testing
- Various assistive devices for evaluating ADL, school, and play-related activities
- Home evaluation for modification and assistive device/equipment recommendation

Standardized Tests
- Wee Functional Independence Measure (Wee FIM^{SM})
- Miller Assessment for preschoolers (MAP)
- Peabody Developmental Motor Scales
- Battelle Developmental Inventory
- Vineland Adaptive Behavior Scales-Revised
- Functional Independence Measure (FIM^{SM})
- Barthel Index
- Play History

Prognosis and Outcome

DMD is a progressive disorder. As the disease progresses, the person with DMD often dies of respiratory difficulties due to dystrophy of respiratory muscles. The primary desired outcome is to maintain ADL independence and function as long as possible with or without the use of assistive technology and/or environmental adaptations. Family counseling and adjustment may be needed in the process of coping with the progression of the disease.

eating disorders: anorexia nervosa/bulimia nervosa

Anorexia nervosa is characterized by the individual's refusal to maintain "a minimally normal body weight, intense fear of gaining weight, and exhibition of a significant disturbance in the perception of the shape or size of the body" (Reed, 2001, p. 779). Central features of bulimia nervosa are binge eating and inappropriate compensatory methods to prevent weight gain, including self-induced vomiting. "To qualify for the diagnosis, the binge eating and inappropriate compensatory behaviors must occur, on average, at least twice a week for three months" (American Psychiatric Association, 1994).

Etiology

Anorexia Nervosa

Onset usually occurs in early to late adolescence, but has been documented in the 20s. The disorder is primarily seen in females (95%), though when seen in males, it generally presents itself in preadolescence (Beers & Berkow, 1999). The cause is unclear, and the literature reveals many explanations, including:

- Psychological issues
- Cognitive distortions
- Dysfunctional families
- Social pressure
- Learned behavior
- Physiologic disturbances

Bulimia nervosa

Males and females are affected, though the typical case is a female in her mid-20s. The precise etiology is unknown for this disorder. There are predisposing features that have been identified in the literature:

- Mood swings
- Impaired family dynamics
- Impulsivity
- Lack of internal control
- High anxiety
- Low self-esteem

Symptoms

Anorexia Nervosa (American Psychiatric Association, 1994)

- Refusal to maintain body weight at or above a minimally normal weight for age and height
- Intense fear of gaining weight or becoming fat, even though underweight
- Disturbance in the manner in which one's body weight or shape is experienced, undue influence of body weight or shape on self-evaluation, or denial of the seriousness of the current low body weight
- In post-menarcheal females, amenorrhea (absence of at least three consecutive menstrual cycles

Bulimia Nervosa (American Psychiatric Association, 1994)

- Recurrent episodes of binge eating
- Recurrent inappropriate compensatory behavior in order to prevent weight gain
- The binge eating and inappropriate compensatory behaviors both occur on average at least twice per week for three months

- Self-evaluation is unduly influenced by body weight and shape
- The disturbance does not occur exclusively during episodes of anorexia nervosa

Assessment Objectives

The occupational therapist will be responsible for assessing occupational performance areas and components. All areas assessed will be considered in relation to functional performance. Key areas for assessment include various performance areas and skills in order to identify realistic client-centered treatment goals.

Assessment of Performance Areas

- Activities of daily living: BADL and IADL skills
- Home Management skills
- Play or Leisure Activities
- Work or Job Performance skills

Assessment of Performance Components

Neuromusculoskeletal

- Range of motion
- Strength
- Endurance

Motor

- Gross coordination

Cognitive Integration and Cognitive Components

- Attention span
- Initiation of activity
- Problem solving

Psychosocial Skills

- Interests
- Self-concept
- Interpersonal skills
- Self-expression
- Coping
- Self-control

Standardized Assessment Tools

- Activity Record
- Functional Capacity Evaluation Battery
- Occupational Case Analysis and Interview Rating Scale (OCAIRS)

- Functional Independence Measure v. 4.0 (FIM^{SM})
- Assessment of Motor and Process Skills (AMPS)

Prognosis and Outcome

An individual may be able to regain independence in daily function and occupational roles.

Erb's palsy See brachial plexus injury.

fetal alcohol syndrome

Fetal alcohol syndrome (FAS) is due to maternal alcohol abuse during pregnancy. The most serious consequence is severe mental retardation due to impaired brain development. Severely affected newborns have growth retardation and are microcephalic (Beers & Berkow, 1999).

Etiology

FAS has been diagnosed in neonates born to chronic alcoholic mothers who drank throughout their pregnancies. Lesser degrees of alcohol abuse result in a less severe manifestation of FAS termed fetal alcohol effect (FAE). Maternal alcohol abuse during pregnancy is considered to be the most common cause of drug-induced teratogenesis. Damage can occur in various regions of the brain. The areas that might be affected by alcohol exposure depend on which areas are developing at the time the alcohol is consumed. The regions of the brain that are most seriously affected by prenatal alcohol exposure in terms of ability to function are: corpus callosum, hippocampus, hypothalamus, basal ganglia, and the frontal lobes.

Rates of FAS are higher in North America than in other countries. The incidence of FAS is highest among American Indians, blacks, and individuals of low socioeconomic status.

Symptoms

Most infants with FAS are irritable, do not eat well, are extra-sensitive to sensory stimulation, and have a strong startle reflex. They may hyperextend their heads or limbs, and can exhibit hypertonia, hypotonia, or both. Some infants may have heart defects or suffer anomalies to the ears, eyes, liver, or joints. Most children with FAS have developmental delays and some have lower than normal IQ. The extent of physiological characteristics tends to correspond with the degree of developmental delays. Most children with FAS have IQs that are legally considered in the normal range.

The most serious characteristics of FAS are the so-called invisible symptoms of neurological damage that results from prenatal exposure to alcohol. These symptoms include:

- Attention deficits
- Memory deficits
- Hyperactivity
- Difficulty with abstract concepts (math, time, money)
- Poor problem-solving skills
- Difficulty learning from consequences
- Poor judgment
- Immature behavior
- Poor impulse control

Adults with FAS have difficulty maintaining successful independence. They have trouble staying in school, keeping jobs, and sustaining healthy interpersonal relationships. Individuals with FAS and related disorders often have symptoms or behavior issues that are a direct result of damage to the prefrontal cortex, which is the part of the brain that controls "executive functions." The executive functions of the prefrontal cortex include:

- Inhibition
- Planning
- Time perception
- Internal ordering
- Working memory
- Self-monitoring
- Verbal self-regulation
- Motor control
- Regulation of emotion
- Motivation

Assessment Objectives

The OT will be responsible for assessing performance areas and components. Performance components essential for BADL function within the child's various environments, cognition and problem solving, and determination of informal caregiver support are all prime assessment domains to explore in order to identify realistic client-centered treatment goals.

Assessment of Performance Areas

- Activities of daily living: BADL and simple IADL skills
- Work and productive activities: safety procedures, educational, prevocational, and vocational
- Play/leisure activities

Assessment of Performance Components

Sensory Processing

- Tactile
- Proprioceptive
- Vestibular
- Visual
- Auditory
- Olfactory
- Gustatory

Perceptual Processing

- Stereognosis
- Kinesthesia
- Pain response
- Body scheme
- Right-left discrimination
- Form constancy
- Position in space
- Visual closure
- Figure ground
- Depth perception
- Spatial relations
- Topographical orientation

Neuromusculoskeletal

- Reflex
- Range of motion
- Muscle tone
- Strength
- Endurance
- Postural control
- Postural alignment

Motor

- Gross coordination
- Crossing the midline

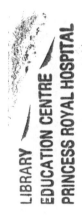

- Laterality
- Bilateral integration
- Motor control
- Praxis
- Fine coordination/dexterity
- Visual-motor integration
- Oral-motor control

Cognitive Integration and Cognitive Components

- Level of arousal
- Orientation
- Recognition
- Attention span
- Initiation of activity
- Termination of activity
- Memory and sequencing
- Spatial operations
- Problem solving
- Learning
- Generalization

Psychosocial Skills

- Interests
- Self-concept
- Social conduct
- Interpersonal skills
- Self-expression
- Coping
- Self-control
- Role performance

Standardized Assessment Tools

- DeGangi-Berk Test of Sensory Integration (DBTSI)
- Test of Sensory Functions in Infants (TSFI)
- Sensory Integration and Praxis Tests
- Bayley Scales of Infant Development-II (BSID-II)
- The Beery-Buktenica Developmental Test of Visual-Motor Integration (VMI-4), 4th ed.
- Bruininks-Oseretsky Test of Motor Proficiency (BOTMP)
- Peabody Developmental Motor Scales
- Test of Visual-Motor Skills—Revised (TVMS—R)

- Test of Visual-Perceptual Skills (non-motor)—Revised
- Tennessee Self-Concept Scale—Revised

Prognosis and Outcome

The person with fetal alcohol syndrome may always require a supervised and assisted living environment (Reed, 2001). The degree to which the individual will be able to live independently will be determined by the extent of the symptoms. Alcohol exposure appears to damage some parts of the brain, while sparing others. Some individuals will have evidence of neurological damage in a few parts of the brain, while others have damage in several regions. Their behavior problems should be viewed with respect to neurological dysfunction. Although psychological factors such as abuse and neglect can exacerbate behavior problems in FAS, one must view the behaviors as primarily organic in origin.

Guillain-Barré syndrome

Guillain-Barré syndrome (GBS) is a rapidly progressive lower motor neuron disorder characterized by muscle weakness and mild sensory loss (Beers & Berkow, 1999). GBS often begins a few days or weeks following an infection, surgery, or immunization. Demyelination or axonal degeneration occurs in the peripheral nerves, spinal nerves, or certain cranial nerves. The most prominent symptom is muscle weakness. The person might also have some sensory impairments. The person's functional skills are affected depending on the muscles involved. Respiratory failure can occur in a small number of cases. GBS is also called Landry's ascending paralysis, infectious polyneuritis, or polyradiculoneuritis.

Etiology

The exact cause is unknown but it is thought to be a viral infection compromising the immune system, resulting in inflammation and degeneration of the peripheral nervous system.

Symptoms

Common symptoms include muscle weakness of various parts of the body and sensory involvement in the distal parts of the body and extremities. Loss of self-care skills and functional independence occur due to muscle weakness and loss of function.

Assessment Objectives

The OT will be responsible for assessing occupational performance areas and components. All areas assessed will be considered in relation to functional performance. Key areas for assessment include various performance areas and skills in order to identify realistic client-centered treatment goals.

Assessment of Performance Areas

- Activities of daily living: BADL and simple IADL skills
- Play and leisure skills
- Work/productivity skills

Assessment of Performance Components

Sensory Processing
- Proprioceptive
- Tactile

Perceptual Processing
- Stereognosis
- Kinesthesia
- Position in space

Neuromusculoskeletal
- Range of motion
- Muscle tone
- Strength
- Endurance
- Postural control
- Soft tissue integrity

Motor
- Gross coordination
- Bilateral integration
- Motor control
- Praxis
- Fine coordination/dexterity
- Oral-motor control

Cognitive Integration
- Attention span
- Memory
- Initiation of activity
- Problem solving

- Learning
- Generalization

Psychosocial Skills/Psychological Components

- Values
- Interests
- Self-concept
- Role performance
- Self-expression

Standardized Assessment Tools

- ADL scales
- Occupational performance history
- Work history, job analysis review
- Leisure activities checklist
- Manual Muscle Test (withheld during acute stages of recovery)
- Range of Motion Test (ROM)
- Sensory Testing
- Home evaluation for modification and assistive device/equipment recommendation

Standardized Tests

- Functional Independence Measure (FIM^SM)
- Barthel Index
- Modified Interest Checklist
- Occupational Performance History Interview
- Jebson Hand function test

Prognosis and Outcome

The prognosis is generally good, with about 95% of the individuals recovering completely within 2 years. The remaining 5% have various residual limitations resulting from muscle weakness.

The primary desired outcome is improving or maintaining muscle strength, endurance, range of motion, ADL skills, and work and leisure skills. Assistive devices or environmental modifications may be necessary to optimize functional independence. Training family members in appropriate assistance of the client may be necessary.

hand injuries

Hand injuries include the loss of functional abilities and sensation in the hand. The human hand is extremely versatile, has multiple functions, and is vital to human function and appearance. It is a major organ of sensation, allowing feeling without looking and protection for injury. The hand is a tool of emotional expression, a communication device for the deaf and the eye of the visually handicapped. The incidence of upper extremity injuries accounts for about a third of all injuries (Kasch, 1996).

Etiology

The causes include amputation of any part of the hand, tendon injuries, nerve injuries, joint dislocation, joint deformity, cumulative trauma disorders, contractures, and fractures.

Symptoms

The primary symptoms in general are:

- Change in posture of the hand
- Pain including numbness and tingling
- Edema
- Limitations in joint range (due to tightness, contracture, or deformity)
- Muscle weakness
- Loss of sensation—touch, pressure, localization and proprioception, temperature and vibration, and stereognosis
- Hand function deficits—grip, grasp, manipulation, dexterity, and bilateral coordination
- Skin changes—color and condition

Assessment Objectives

The occupational therapist will be responsible for assessing occupational performance areas and components. Hand therapy is most beneficial and essential for optimal results during the restorative phase following the initial physiological wound healing. All areas assessed will be considered in relation to functional performance. Key areas for assessment include various performance areas and skills in order to identify realistic client-centered treatment goals.

Assessment of Performance Areas

- Activities of daily living: BADL and simple IADL skills
- Play and leisure skills
- School/educational setting if applicable
- Work/productivity skills

Assessment of Performance Components

Sensory Processing
- Proprioceptive
- Tactile

Perceptual Processing
- Stereognosis
- Kinesthesia

Neuromusculoskeletal
- Range of motion
- Strength
- Endurance
- Soft tissue integrity

Motor
- Gross coordination
- Bilateral integration
- Motor control
- Praxis
- Fine coordination/dexterity
- Laterality

Cognitive Integration
- Attention span
- Memory
- Problem solving
- Learning
- Generalization

Psychosocial Skills/Psychological Components
- Interests

Standardized Assessment Tools

- Goniometer, Dynamometer, Pinch meter
- Circumferential or volumetric measurement of edema
- Manual muscle test
- Hand function test
- Sensory testing
- ADL scales
- Home and environmental evaluation
- Occupational performance history
- Leisure activities checklist

Standardized Tests
- Functional Independence Measure (FIM^{SM})
- Barthel Index
- Minnesota Rate of Manipulation Test (MRMT)
- Minnesota Manual Dexterity Test (MMDT)
- Jebson Hand function test
- Purdue Pegboard
- McGill Pain Questionnaire (MPQ)
- Modified Interest Checklist
- Occupational Performance History Interview
- Worker Role Inventory

Prognosis and Outcome

Prognosis varies depending on the severity of the injury, intensity of hand therapy, and limitations presented by coexisting medical diagnoses. The outcome of hand therapy also depends on the cognition, learning skills, and motivation of the individual, notably in hand function reeducation programs. Usually the conditions improve with medical and surgical intervention, hand therapy supplemented and continued with home program, splinting, and activity modifications. Complete recovery to normalcy may not be achievable in all cases.

hip fracture/hip arthroplasty

Fractures of the femoral neck are classified as occult, impact, displaced, or non-displaced. The person presents with groin pain and a shortened, externally rotated leg that is painful to move. Compromised blood supply can seriously impede healing, which may lead to osteonecrosis and non-union (Beers & Berkow, 1999).

There are five common sites of femoral fractures. Three occur at the neck: subcapital, transcervical, and basilar. The fourth occurs at the intertrochanter, called intertrochanteric, and the fifth site is in the shaft below the trochanters, called subtrochanteric.

Fractures of the intertrochanter are classified by the number of bony fragments and by the inherent instability. Two, three, and four part fractures have been described. Blood supply is usually maintained and osteonecrosis and non-union are more seldom seen than with femoral neck fractures. Hip arthroplasty is the surgical replacement formation, or reformation of the hip joint (Gower & Bowker, 1993).

Etiology

The most common cause of hip fracture is trauma caused by a fall, sudden rotational force, or impact as might be sustained in a motor vehicle accident. Degeneration of the head of the femur, due to necrosis or loss of bone strength and density as in osteoporosis and osteoarthritis, enhances the risk of a fracture. Open reduction internal fixation (ORIF) is a common surgical intervention with intertrochanteric and subtrochanteric fractures. Incidence rates of fracture are greater for women than men. Partial or total hip replacements (arthroplasty/THR/THA) are most frequently done when pain from osteoarthritis adversely affects ADL and functional mobility status. THR and partial-THR may also be done following hip fracture and other disease processes.

Hip fractures in the elderly represent a significant threat to well-being. Depending upon the study, the mortality rate of hip fracture patients may be as high as 25% (Wolinsky, 1997). Estimates of recovery after fracture have suggested that anywhere from 25% to 75% of these individuals will not achieve their pre-morbid level of function (Magaziner, Simonside, Kasher, Hebel, & Kenzora,1990). Poor recovery is associated with older age, pre-fracture dependency, longer hospital stay, dementia, post-surgical delirium in patients without dementia, and lack of contact with a social support system (Mutran, Reitzes, Mossey, Fernandez, & Erlinder, 1998).

Symptoms

Several factors shape assessment intervention. These include the type of surgery (THR or ORIF) and the surgeon's preference regarding post-surgical precautions. Precautions usually include but are not limited to:

• Non–weight-bearing to partial weight bearing 6 weeks or longer
• Limited hip flexion, external rotation, abduction, adduction, extension, and internal rotation

This information is usually available in the medical record or may require direct communication with the surgeon.

Assessment Objectives

The OT will be responsible for assessing occupational perform-ance areas and components. All areas assessed will be considered in relation to functional performance. Key areas for assessment include various performance areas and skills in order to identify realistic client-centered treatment goals.

Assessment of Performance Areas

- Activities of daily living: BADL and IADL skills
- Vocational skills
- Home management
- Play/leisure

Assessment of Performance Components

Sensory Processing
- Proprioceptive
- Vestibular
- Visual

Perceptual Processing
- Kinesthesia
- Position in space
- Figure ground
- Body scheme
- Depth perception
- Spatial relations
- Topographical orientation

Neuromusculoskeletal
- Range of motion
- Strength
- Endurance
- Postural control
- Postural alignment
- Soft tissue integrity

Motor
- Gross coordination
- Motor control
- Praxis
- Visual-motor integration

Cognitive Integration
- Orientation
- Attention span
- Memory
- Sequencing
- Initiation of activity

- Termination of activity
- Spatial operations
- Problem solving
- Learning
- Generalization

Psychosocial Skills/Psychological Components

- Interests
- Self-concept
- Role performance

Standardized Assessment Tools

- Manual Muscle Test (MMT)
- Range of Motion test (AROM and PROM)
- Pain Scales (Numeric or Verbal Rating)
- Klein-Bell ADL Scale
- Functional Independence Measure, version 4 (FIM^{SM})
- Berg Balance Test
- Tinetti Test of Balance and Gait
- Rhomberg Test of Balance
- Sensory Testing
- Self-Esteem Scale
- Geriatric Depression Scale
- Self-Assessment of Leisure Interests
- Occupational Therapy Home Evaluation
- Goniometer

Prognosis and Outcome

Recovery may require up to six months, with the typical case requiring 2–3 months. A person who is independent prior to hip repair surgery should be independent after surgery. Successful outcomes include: relief of pain, maintenance of a good position of the fracture, allowance for bony union for fracture healing, and restoration of optimal function to the person.

HIV (human immunodeficiency virus), AIDS (acquired immunodeficiency syndrome)

Human immunodeficiency virus (HIV) was first identified in 1983 by French scientist Luc Montagnier (O'Dell & Dillon, 1996). The HIV is a retrovirus (Lentivirus family) that destroys CD_4 T-cells (helper Ts), white blood cells responsible for activating the immune system's natural disease-fighting mechanism (Newman, Echevarria, & Digman, 1995). The virus has a long latency period and has a direct primary destructive effect on various body tissues. The central and peripheral nervous systems are also damaged when HIV invades the neuronal cells. The secondary disorders include opportunistic infections such as *Pneumocystis carinii* pneumonia, *Candida albicans*, *Cryptococcus neoformans*, *Toxoplasma gondii*, cytomegalovirus, mycobacterium avium-intracellular complex, or *Mycobacterium tuberculosis* and malignancies such as Karposi's sarcoma. Additional disorders include polyneuropathy, radiculopathy, segmental demyelination, and ganglioneuronitis.

Etiology

The cause of acquired immunodeficiency syndrome is the human immunodeficiency virus, which appears in two major forms (HIV-1 and HIV-2). HIV is transmitted by intimate sexual contact, exposure to infected blood or blood products, body fluids containing infected cells with lymphocytes or plasma, and perinatal transmission from mother to fetus. The groups most affected are sexually active homosexual and bisexual men, intravenous drug users, and hemophiliacs infected by blood transfusions. Persons with CD_4 T-cells (helper Ts) count below 200/mL meet the definition of AIDS, regardless of clinical symptomatology.

Symptoms

HIV infection is noted to have 4 stages:

- Stage 1: Acute infection—acute viral syndrome with fever, sweats, nausea, diarrhea, and pharyngitis
- Stage 2: Asymptomatic disease—relative viral latency, range of 1–15 years
- Stage 3: Symptomatic HIV—CD_4 T-cells (helper Ts) count below 500/mL, generalized persistent lymphadenopathy
- Stage 4: Advanced HIV disease or acquired immunodeficiency syndrome—the more familiar clinical manifestations occur with severely compromised immune system. Symptoms progress from mild weakness to disability at variable rates, with respiratory issues, pain, cognitive dysfunction, communication disorders, dysphagia, loss of functional abilities to total dependence.

Assessment Objectives

The OT will be responsible for assessing occupational performance areas and components. It has to be noted that in the symptomatic and later stages the rapid and frequent medical and functional status changes require frequent reassessments. All areas assessed will be considered in relation to functional performance. Key areas for assessment include various performance areas and skills in order to identify realistic client-centered treatment goals.

Assessment of Performance Areas

- Activities of daily living: BADL and IADL skills
- Home management skills
- Work/productivity skills
- Play and leisure skills
- School/educational setting if applicable

Assessment of Performance Components

Sensory Processing
- Proprioceptive
- Tactile
- Vestibular
- Visual
- Auditory

Perceptual Processing
- Stereognosis
- Kinesthesia
- Position in space
- Body scheme
- Depth perception
- Spatial relations
- Topographical orientation

Neuromusculoskeletal
- Range of motion
- Muscle tone
- Strength
- Endurance
- Postural control
- Soft tissue integrity

Motor
- Gross coordination
- Bilateral integration
- Motor control
- Praxis
- Fine coordination/dexterity
- Visual-motor integration
- Oral-motor control

Cognitive Integration
- Level of arousal
- Orientation
- Recognition
- Attention span
- Memory
- Sequencing
- Spatial operations
- Problem solving
- Learning
- Generalization

Psychosocial Skills/Psychological Components
- Values
- Interests
- Self-concept
- Role performance
- Interpersonal skills
- Self-expression

Standardized Assessment Tools

- ADL scales
- Occupational performance history
- Work history, job analysis review
- Leisure activities checklist
- Manual Muscle Test
- Range of Motion test (ROM)
- Sensory Testing
- Home Evaluation for modification and assistive device/equipment recommendation

Standardized Tests
- Functional Independence Measure (FIM^{SM})
- Barthel Index

- Modified Interest Checklist
- Occupational Performance History Interview
- Jebson Hand Function Test
- Pizzi Assessment of Productive Living for Adults with HIV Infection and AIDS (PAPL)
- McGill Pain Questionnaire (MPQ)

Prognosis and Outcome

The prognosis for individuals with full-blown AIDS is poor. The use of multi-drug therapy has prolonged survival. Patients eventually succumb to opportunistic infections. With advances in medical management and drugs and resultant increased survival rate, more people are learning to live with a chronic disease. Desired outcomes include: improving or maintaining muscle strength, endurance, range of motion, ADL skills, and work and leisure skills. Assistive devices or environmental modifications may be necessary to optimize functional independence. Training of caretakers and family members in appropriate assistance of the client is absolutely necessary.

homelessness

According to the Stewart B. McKinney Act, a person is considered homeless if he or she lacks a fixed, regular, and adequate night-time residence; if he or she has a primary night-time residence that is publicly supervised or privately operated with the intention that it is to be used as a temporary living accommodation and/or temporary residence for individuals intended to be institutionalized; or if he or she utilizes a public or private place not typically used as a regular sleeping accommodation for human beings. Homelessness is a sociocultural term. It is largely an urban phenomenon; 71% of the homeless are from urban areas (National Resource Center on Homelessness and Mental Illness).

The government only collects statistics on those homeless people who have applied to local authorities for help—usually families with children and others deemed to be especially vulnerable. Government figures, therefore, do not include overall figures on the number of single homeless people. Homelessness has increased significantly in recent years. This has been due to a number of economic and social factors, including the decline of availability in rented accommodation, lack of affordable accommodation for those on low incomes, rising unemployment, and the growth in single households.

There are several stages of homelessness. *Marginally homeless* refers to individuals who live near poverty level and utilize community resources such as food and clothing pantries. *Recently homeless* refers to individuals who may or may not consider themselves homeless, but have many needs that center around locating and utilizing resources that aim to diminish their health and social needs. *Chronically homeless* refers to individuals who accept their homeless lifestyle and do not seek out services, but receive assistance when outreach workers approach them (Belcher, Scholler-Jacquish, & Drummond, 1991).

Many people who experience homelessness also experience physical disability or mental illness (mental illness is common in 20–25% of the homeless), and OT seems to be a natural fit to meet the needs of this diverse group of people. Community rehabilitation is a well-known aspect of social development addressing the health issues at the community level, through intervention focused around the client's particular point of need.

Etiology

There are varied and complex reasons as to why people become homeless.

- Poverty: lack of livable income
- Housing: expensive housing and decline in the number of affordable housing units
- Disability: the disabled are unable to work and must rely on entitlements such as SSI; in this situation one can find it almost impossible to maintain reasonable housing
- Untreated mental illness: impossible to maintain employment, pay bills, or keep supportive social relationships
- Substance abuse and co-occurring disorders
- Other circumstances include domestic violence, unexpected health care expenses, post incarceration, divorce, and so on

Symptoms

- Lack of housing or an address
- Lack of livable income—part-time employed, very poorly paid or unemployed
- Poor hygiene, deficient or lack of self-care skills
- Poor self-esteem, lack of social skills

- Deficits in money, time-management skills, problem solving, coping and adaptive strategies
- Health and mental wellness issues

Assessment Objectives

The OT will be responsible for assessing occupational performance areas and components. All areas assessed will be considered in relation to functional performance. Key areas for assessment include various performance areas and skills in order to identify realistic client-centered treatment goals.

Assessment of Performance Areas

- Activities of daily living: BADL and simple IADL skills
- Social activities and leisure skills
- Work/productivity skills
- School/educational setting if applicable

Assessment of Performance Components

Cognitive Integration
- Problem solving
- Learning
- Generalization

Psychosocial Skills/Psychological Components
- Values
- Interests
- Self-concept
- Social conduct
- Role performance
- Interpersonal skills
- Self-control
- Self-expression

Standardized Assessment Tools

Homelessness is complex with a combination of several areas of concern. Assessment tools have to fit into the context of the individual's needs and additionally have significant and immediate meaning to the client's goals. In practice, the tools need to be relevant to the setup limits and conditions of the evaluation site. Non-standardized and/or standardized tests may be used depending on the acute relevancy of the tests.

- ADL scales
- Occupational performance history
- Leisure activities checklist
- Work history
- Cognitive and perceptual evaluation scales

Standardized Tests
- Modified Interest Checklist
- Occupational Performance History Interview
- Self-Esteem Scale
- Worker Role Inventory
- Allen Cognitive Level Test
- Kohlman Evaluation of Living Skills (KELS)
- Social Readjustment Rating Scale

Prognosis and Outcome

The homeless individual with a true motivation to becoming self-sufficient and independent has excellent potential for positive change in his or her lifestyle with well-guided and structured use of state, federal, and local private homeless assistance programs for food, shelter, workshops, education, and vocational training.

hyperactive child syndrome See attention deficit/hyperactive disorder (ADHD).

hyperkinetic impulse disorder See attention deficit/hyperactive disorder (ADHD).

Klumpke's palsy See brachial plexus injury.

learning disabilities

Learning disabilities are neurological disorders that interfere with a person's ability to store, process, or produce information, and create a gap between one's ability and performance. Individuals with learning disabilities are generally of average or above average intelligence. Learning disabilities encompass cognitive problems in acquiring daily living, social, language, or communication and academic skills (Duran & Fisher, 1999). Sometimes overlooked as hidden handicaps, learning disabilities are often not easily recognized, accepted, or considered serious once detected. Learning disabilities affect children and adults. The impact of the disability ranges from relatively mild to severe (National Center for Learning Disabilities, 1999). Depending on how learning disorders are defined, up to 60% of ADHD children have a coexisting learning disorder (CHADD, 2001). Dyslexia, dysgraphia, dyscalculia, dyspraxia/apraxia, auditory discrimination, and visual perceptual deficits are common symptoms of learning disabilities.

According to *DSM-IV-TR,* "Learning disorders are diagnosed when the individual's achievement on individually administered, standardized tests in reading, mathematics, or written expression is substantially below that expected for age, schooling, and level of intelligence" (American Psychiatric Association, 2000, p. 49).

Etiology

The precise cause of learning disabilities is not known. Learning disabilities are presumed to be disorders of the central nervous system and a variety of factors may contribute to their occurrence.

- Heredity: Learning disabilities tend to run in families.
- Problems during pregnancy and childbirth: Illness or injury during or before birth may cause learning disabilities. Learning disabilities may also be caused by the use of drugs and alcohol during pregnancy, RH incompatibility with the mother (if untreated), premature or prolonged labor or lack of oxygen, or low weight at birth.
- Incidents after birth: Head injuries, nutritional deprivation, poisonous substances, (e.g., lead), and child abuse can contribute to learning disabilities.

Symptoms

Delayed or atypical development can be notable in children with learning disabilities. However, parents and teachers should not make hasty judgments because developmental variations exist among all children. However, observation and specific professional evaluation needs to be done on behaviors for a clear diagnosis and appropriate timely and efficient intervention.

Examples of at-risk behaviors include:

- Language: Slow development of speech; difficulty learning new vocabulary or naming familiar items; use of two or three word phrases instead of strings of words; speech is difficult to understand; difficulty expressing wants or needs; trouble following even simple directions.

- Motor: Difficulty manipulating small objects (using pencil/crayon); poor balance; awkwardness with jumping, running, or climbing; poor sense of personal space
- Sensory: Loss of vision, hearing, touch, proprioception, taste, or smell may also exist. These are usually detected in the earlier stages of development and significantly influence all other activities and behaviors.
- Social: Difficulty with (or disinterest in) peer socialization; overly aggressive or withdrawn; sudden and extreme mood changes; frequent crying or tantrums; poor frustration tolerance.
- Cognitive: Difficulty understanding cause and effect; problems with sequencing and one-to-one correspondence; difficulty with basic concepts (size, shape, and color)
- Self-help: Difficulty with washing, dressing, self-feeding
- Attention: Easily distracted, acts impulsively, displays poor organizational skills

Assessment Objectives

The OT will be responsible for assessing occupational performance areas and components that affect independence in areas of personal, social, academic, and vocational pursuits. All areas assessed will be considered in relation to functional performance. Key areas for assessment include various performance areas and skills in order to identify realistic client-centered treatment goals.

Assessment of Performance Areas

- Activities of daily living: BADL and simple IADL skills
- Play and leisure skills
- School/educational setting if applicable
- Work/productivity skills

Assessment of Performance Components

Sensory Processing

- Proprioceptive
- Tactile
- Vestibular
- Visual
- Auditory
- Gustatory
- Olfactory

Perceptual Processing
- Stereognosis
- Kinesthesia
- Position in space
- Right-left discrimination
- Form constancy
- Visual closure
- Figure ground
- Body scheme
- Depth perception
- Spatial relations
- Topographical orientation

Neuromusculoskeletal
- Muscle tone
- Endurance
- Postural control

Motor
- Gross coordination
- Bilateral integration
- Motor control
- Praxis
- Fine coordination/dexterity
- Laterality
- Crossing the midline
- Visual-motor integration
- Oral-motor control

Cognitive Integration
- Recognition
- Attention span
- Memory
- Sequencing
- Categorization
- Initiation of activity
- Termination of activity
- Concept formation
- Spatial operations
- Problem solving
- Learning
- Generalization

Psychosocial Skills/Psychological Components
- Interests
- Self-concept
- Social conduct
- Role performance
- Interpersonal skills
- Self-control
- Self-expression

Standardized Assessment Tools
- ADL scales
- Developmental scales
- Hand function tests
- Play scales
- Cognitive and perceptual tests

Standardized Tests
- Assessment of Motor and Process Skills (AMPS)
- Developmental Test of Visual Perception, 2nd Edition (DTVP-2)
- Children's Playfulness Scale
- Play Observation
- Peabody Developmental Motor Scales (PDMS)
- Functional Independence Measure (FIM^{SM})
- Crawford Small Parts Dexterity Test (1981 Revised)
- Sensory Integration and Praxis Tests (SIPT)
- Vineland Adaptive Behavior Scales-Revised (VABS-R)

Prognosis and Outcome

Learning disabilities can be lifelong conditions. In some people, several overlapping learning disabilities may be apparent. Other people may have a single, isolated learning problem that has little impact on their lives. Specially trained educators may perform a diagnostic educational evaluation assessing the child's academic and intellectual potential and level of academic performance. Building on the child's abilities and strengths while correcting and compensating for disabilities and weaknesses will contribute to a better outcome. Speech and language programs and psychological services also may be incorporated. Some medications may be effective in helping the child learn by enhancing attention and concentration.

limb-girdle muscular dystrophy

Limb-girdle muscular dystrophy is one of an inherited group of at least 10 different muscular dystrophies that initially affects the muscles of the shoulder girdle and the hips. The disease is progressive and may involve other muscles over a period of time.

Etiology

Typically, onset includes pelvic muscle weakness (difficulty standing from a sitting position without using arms, climbing stairs) in childhood to young adulthood. Later there is the onset of shoulder weakness with progression to significant loss of mobility or wheelchair dependence over the next 20–30 years.

Symptoms

- Muscle weakness in the pelvis, hips, upper legs, shoulders
- Loss of muscle mass in the same areas (atrophy)
- Abnormal, sometimes waddling walking gait
- Later in the disease there can be facial muscle weakness
- Later in the disease muscles of the lower legs, feet, lower arms, and hands can become weak
- Late in the disease there can be contractures of joints
- Palpitations or passing out spells can develop from abnormal heart rhythms
- Sometimes the calves will appear large and muscular (pseudo-hypertrophy), but are actually not strong

Assessment Objectives

The OT will be responsible for assessing occupational performance areas and components. All areas assessed will be considered in relation to functional performance. Key areas for assessment include various performance areas and skills in order to identify realistic client-centered treatment goals.

Assessment of Performance Areas

- Activities of daily living: BADL and IADL skills
- Work and productive activities
- Vocational Activities: Work or job performance
- Home management
- Play or leisure activities

Assessment of Performance Components

Perceptual Processing
- Kinesthesia
- Position in space
- Spatial relations
- Topographical orientation

Neuromusculoskeletal
- Reflexes
- Range of motion
- Muscle tone
- Strength
- Endurance
- Postural alignment
- Postural control

Motor
- Gross coordination
- Bilateral integration
- Motor control, praxis, and fine coordination/dexterity

Cognitive Integration and Cognitive Components
- Attention span
- Problem solving
- Sequencing
- Learning
- Generalization

Psychosocial Skills
- Interests
- Self-concept
- Interpersonal skills
- Self-expression
- Coping
- Self-control
- Time management

Standardized Assessment Tools

- Functional Independence Measure v.4.0 (FIM^{SM})
- Assessment of Motor and Process Skills (AMPS), 2nd ed.
- Manual Muscle test (MMT)
- Range of Motion test (AROM and PROM)
- Pain Scales (Numeric or Verbal Rating)

- Klein-Bell ADL Scale
- Berg Balance Test
- Tinetti Test of Balance and Gait
- Rhomberg Test of Balance
- Sensory Testing
- Self-Esteem Scale
- Geriatric Depression Scale
- Self-Assessment of Leisure Interests
- Occupational Therapy Home Evaluation
- The Interest Checklist
- Goniometry
- Dynamometer
- Pinch Meter

Prognosis and Outcome

It is to be generally understood that it is expected that there will be slow progression of weakness. In addition, as the disease progresses, slowly more muscles or parts of the body become weak. Of particular concern is heart muscle weakness and a tendency to have abnormal electrical activity of the heart. This can increase the risk of palpitations, falling out, and sudden death. Most patients with this group of diseases live into adulthood, but do not reach their full life expectancy (Muscular Dystrophy Association, 2001).

low back pain

Low back pain may be accompanied by pain radiating down the buttocks and legs in the distribution of the sciatic nerve called sciatica. Regional back pain may be specific to the back area, which may include pain related to sprain, injury to muscles and ligaments, and spondylosis. Radicular pain refers to pain in the leg and back related to nerve root irritation. Excessive or prolonged nerve irritation and the extent of involvement may lead to muscle weakness and sensory loss.

Etiology

There are various factors that cause low back pain. Sprain to the ligaments and strain to muscles cause localized back pain. Chronic conditions that cause back pain include osteoarthritis, ankylosing spondylitis to the lumbosacral areas, and chronic muscle and ligament injuries. Back pain also results from nerve involvement in the spinal column resulting in pain in and around the muscles supplied by the nerves. The prevalence for back pain increases with age and nearly 50% of adults over 60 years report back pain (Larson, 1996; Wilson, Hickey, Gorham, & Childers, 1997).

Symptoms

Symptoms include pain, muscle weakness, sensory loss, limited range resulting from pain and weakness, poor postural control, poor endurance, and poor mobility and ambulation as a result of pain. The person might need assistance for daily activities as a result of inability to move secondary to pain. Pain and weakness may limit a person's ability to do work and involve in leisure related tasks. Pain, weakness, and dependence in daily tasks may lead to depression, anxiety, and other psychological problems.

Assessment Objectives

The OT will be responsible for assessing occupational performance areas and components. The OT will be involved in assessment and management of the following areas throughout the course of the patient's stay in the acute and rehabilitation setting. All areas assessed will be considered in relation to functional performance. Key areas for assessment include various performance areas and skills in order to identify realistic client-centered treatment goals.

Assessment of Performance Areas

- Activities of daily living: BADL and simple IADL skills
- Home management
- Play and leisure skills
- Work/productivity skills

Assessment of Performance Components

Neuromusculoskeletal

- Range of motion
- Muscle tone
- Strength
- Endurance
- Postural control
- Postural alignment

Motor
- Gross coordination
- Motor control

Cognitive Integration
- Problem solving
- Learning
- Generalization

Psychosocial Skills/Psychological Components
- Interests
- Self-concept
- Role performance
- Self-control

Standardized Assessment Tools

- ADL scales
- Occupational performance history
- Work history, job analysis review
- Leisure activities checklist
- Manual Muscle Test (withheld during acute stages of recovery)
- Range of Motion test
- Sensory Testing
- Home Evaluation for modification and assistive device/equipment recommendation
- Depression screening

Standardized Tests
- Functional Independence Measure (FIM^{SM})
- Barthel Index
- Modified Interest Checklist
- Occupational Performance History Interview
- Jebson Hand Function Test
- Beck's depression inventory
- Oswestry Low Back Pain Disability Index
- Coping Strategy Questionnaire
- Pain Disability Index

Prognosis and Outcome

Prognosis varies depending upon the severity of involvement. Often a person may be able to become independent in self-care and work and leisure activities. Modifications may be needed in the physical and social environment to enhance independence.

low vision

The term "low vision" describes a serious visual loss that is uncorrectable by medical or surgical intervention or with eyeglasses (Jose,1983). It is a term used to describe the person's problem, not the underlying pathology or etiology. The term low vision, along with visually impaired, visually handicapped, and partially sighted, implies that a person has some functional vision remaining. A separate term, legally blind, came about in the 1930s, developed by the U.S. federal government to qualify people for certain benefits; 85% of those legally blind have low vision rather than total blindness (Jose,1983).

Etiology

Low vision is defined as bilateral subnormal visual acuity or abnormal visual field resulting from a disorder in the visual system that results in decreased visual performance. Low vision indicates there is a visual impairment severe enough to interfere with the successful performance of activities of daily living, while allowing some usable vision. Low vision is the third most common disability in the United States after arthritis and cardiac disease. Approximately one in six adults who are in the age range of 45-74 and older report moderate to severe visual impairment. Above 75 years of age, the number is one in four. Usually the individual has at least one additional chronic condition (Warren, 1998).

Symptoms

The range of low vision is from 20/80 to 20/1000. Specific problems may include: macular scotoma, ocular pain, blurred vision, diplopia (double vision), distortion of vision, photophobia, flashing lights, halos around lights, abnormal color vision, visual hallucination, night blindness, and inability to discriminate details (Warren, 1998).

Assessment Objectives

The OT will be responsible for assessing occupational performance areas and components. All areas assessed will be considered in relation to functional performance. Key areas for assessment include various performance areas and skills in order to identify realistic client-centered treatment goals.

Assessment of Performance Areas

- Activities of Daily Living: BADL and IADL skills
- Work and productive activities
- Home management
- Vocational and pre-vocational activities
- Play or leisure activities

Assessment of Performance Components

Sensory Processing
- Tactile
- Proprioceptive
- Auditory

Perceptual Processing
- Kinesthesia
- Stereognosis
- Position in space
- Spatial relations
- Depth perception
- Figure ground

Neuromusculoskeletal
- Endurance
- Postural alignment

Motor
- Bilateral integration
- Fine coordination/dexterity
- Visual-motor integration

Cognitive Integration
- Attention span
- Memory
- Sequencing
- Spatial operations
- Problem solving
- Safety and judgment
- Generalization

Psychosocial Skills
- Interests
- Self-concept
- Interpersonal skills
- Coping skills

- Time management
- Self-control

Standardized Assessment Tools

- Functional Independence Measure (FIM[SM])
- Assessment of Motor and Process Skills (AMPS)
- Purdue Pegboard
- Minnesota Low Vision Reading Test
- Assessment for Vision Rehabilitation Services
- Minnesota Spatial Relations Test (MSRT)
- Motor-Free Visual Perception Test-Revised (MVPT-R)
- Motor-Free Visual Perception Test-Vertical (MVPT-V)
- Hooper Visual Organization Test (VOT)
- Leisure Activities Blank
- Interest Checklist

Prognosis and Outcome

Outcome is driven by the individual's willingness and ability to utilize compensatory strategies, environmental adaptations, and assistive technology. It is essential that each person decide which compensatory strategies to use. Each individual will be encouraged to act in his best interest, recognizing diverse levels of motivation.

lymphedema

Lymphedema or lymphatic disease is the abnormal collection of water and protein in the skin and subcutaneous tissues. It is classified as primary or secondary. Primary lymphedema is due to aplastic or hypoplastic lymphatic trunks. Secondary lymphedema occurs with infection and malignant disease (Beers & Berkow, 1999); generally after recurrent infection, tumor, lymphoproliferative disease or injury to the lymphatic system from surgical excision, trauma, or irradiation. Inadequate tissue fluid drainage results in stagnant fluid and proteins, increase in limb girth, higher susceptibility to infection, or cellulitis.

Etiology

Lymphedema develops when the lymphatic load exceeds the transfer capacity of the lymphatic system. Lymphedema can develop several months or years after interruption of the lymphatic pathways following exhaustion of all compensatory mechanisms.

Symptoms

Primary symptoms are:

- Swelling and pain
- Limitations in range of motion
- Loss of self-care skills
- Reduced participation in social and leisure activities

Assessment Objectives

The OT will be responsible for assessing occupational perform-ance areas and components. The OT will be involved in the assess-ment and management throughout the course of the patient's stay in the acute setting, rehabilitation setting, and/or outpatient set-ting. All areas assessed will be considered in relation to functional performance. Key areas for assessment include various perform-ance areas and skills in order to identify realistic client-centered treatment goals.

Assessment of Performance Areas

- Activities of daily living: BADL and IADL skills
- Leisure skills, social activities
- Work/productivity skills

Assessment of Performance Components

Sensory Processing
- Proprioceptive
- Tactile

Perceptual Processing
- Stereognosis
- Kinesthesia
- Position in space

Neuromusculoskeletal
- Range of motion
- Strength
- Endurance
- Postural alignment
- Soft tissue integrity

Motor
- Gross coordination
- Bilateral integration

- Fine coordination/dexterity
- Laterality

Cognitive Integration
- Memory
- Sequencing
- Problem solving
- Learning
- Generalization

Psychosocial Skills/Psychological Components
- Values
- Interests
- Self-concept
- Role performance

Standardized Assessment Tools

- ADL scales
- Circumferential or volumetric measurements of edema
- Range of motion tests
- Hand function evaluation
- Endurance assessment
- Work, home, and leisure activities assessment

Standardized Tests
- Functional Independence Measure (FIM^SM)
- Klein-Bell Activities of Daily Living Scale
- Jebson Hand Function Test
- Modified Interest Checklist
- Occupational Performance History Interview

Prognosis and Outcome

The goals of treatment for lymphedema are to preserve skin integrity, soften subcutaneous tissue, reduce limb size, and avoid contractures. With judicious use of medication to reduce water and protein content and prevention of infection, mechanical compression and/or manual lymph drainage techniques, external volume restriction and surgical intervention (rare and only in a small percentage of patients), edema can be reduced or controlled. Skin care to prevent any infection or injury is very important. Exposure to extreme temperatures should be avoided. Resistive exercise and resting the affected limb are to be avoided. Complete reduction of edema is not always achieved or maintained.

minimal brain dysfunction See attention deficit/hyperactive disorder.

multiple sclerosis

Multiple sclerosis (MS) is a progressive disease of the central nervous system characterized by disseminated patches of demyelination of nerves in scattered areas of the brain and spinal cord that results in multiple and various neurological signs. Exacerbation and remission of the signs and symptoms are typical in multiple sclerosis (Frankel, 1995). In MS the myelin that surrounds the nerve is destroyed and replaced with fibrous tissue that impedes conduction of nerve impulses to and from the brain.

Etiology

The cause of MS is unknown. Various theories exist that suggest various causes such as autoimmune disease, viral disease, trauma, decreased blood flow to the brain, allergies, and genetic susceptibility. The occurrence is more common among women than men and occurs commonly in age groups between 15 and 50 years. In terms of racial predisposition, whites are more affected than other races.

Symptoms

The symptoms depend on the area of the brain and nervous system affected by the disease. For example, if the cerebellum is involved, an individual will present with ataxia and intentional tremor. If the corticospinal tract is involved, a person may show signs of weakness similar to stroke.

Assessment Objectives

The OT will be responsible for assessing occupational performance areas and components. All areas assessed will be considered in relation to functional performance. Key areas for assessment include various performance areas and skills in order to identify realistic client-centered treatment goals.

Assessment of Performance Areas

- Activities of daily living: BADL and IADL skills
- Home management skills
- Play and leisure skills
- Work/productivity skills

Assessment of Performance Components

Sensory Processing
- Proprioceptive
- Tactile
- Vestibular
- Visual

Perceptual Processing
- Stereognosis
- Kinesthesia
- Position in space

Neuromusculoskeletal
- Range of motion
- Muscle tone
- Strength
- Endurance
- Postural control

Motor
- Gross coordination
- Bilateral integration
- Motor control
- Praxis
- Fine coordination/dexterity
- Visual-motor integration
- Oral-motor control

Cognitive Integration
- Orientation
- Attention span
- Memory
- Sequencing
- Initiation of activity
- Termination of activity
- Spatial operations
- Problem solving
- Learning
- Generalization

Psychosocial Skills/Psychological Components
- Values
- Interests

- Self-concept
- Role performance
- Interpersonal skills
- Self-expression
- Time management

Standardized Assessment Tools

- ADL scales
- Occupational performance history
- Work history, job analysis review
- School functional assessment
- Leisure activities checklist
- Muscle Test (goniometer, pinch meter, dynamometer, hand function tests)
- Range of Motion test
- Hand function test in case of the presence of tremor, spasticity, and muscle weakness
- Sensory testing
- Various assistive devices for evaluating ADL, school, and play-related activities
- Home evaluation for modification and assistive device/equipment recommendation

Standardized Tests

- Assessment of Motor and Process Skills, 2nd ed. (AMPS)
- Fatigue Impact Scale (FIS)
- Mini Mental State Examination
- Functional Independence Measure (FIM^SM)
- Barthel Index
- Modified Interest Checklist
- Occupational Performance History Interview
- Jebson Hand function test
- Self-Esteem Scale
- Worker Role Inventory

Prognosis and Outcome

MS is a progressive disease with periods of exacerbations and remissions. The prognosis varies depending on the rate of degeneration and the extent of brain and nerve involvement. The person may be able to maintain a normal lifestyle during periods of remission.

As the person requires more assistance, reassessment of daily skills and retraining of ADL skills with or without assistive devices is needed. As the disease progresses, physical assistance may be needed to maintain daily function, ADL, work, and leisure skills. Environmental modification needs to be done to maintain the quality of life of the individual.

muscular dystrophy See Duchenne's muscular dystrophy and limb-girdle muscular dystrophy.

myasthenia gravis

Myasthenia gravis in adults appears to be an autoimmune disorder. Myasthenia gravis is characterized by episodic muscle weakness caused by loss or dysfunction of acetylcholine receptors at the neuromuscular junction (Beers & Berkow, 1999). It is a chronic progressive, degenerative disorder of striated muscles that lead to weakness in the voluntary muscles. Congenital myasthenia is a rare autosomal recessive disorder of neuromuscular transmission that begins in childhood. Abnormalities in the thymus gland are common in about 75% of affected people (McCormack & Pedretti, 1996). Although it can occur at any age, myasthenia gravis usually appears between the ages of 20 and 30 in women and 50 and 70 in men. Electrodiagnosis with NCS and EMG are used to confirm clinical impression and exclude other disorders in a differential diagnosis (Stolp-Smith, 1996).

Etiology

Myasthenia gravis appears to be an autoimmune disorder in which the body's immune system affects the acetylcholine receptors. It is also thought the condition could be caused by a defect in the resynthesis of acetylcholine on the presynaptic membrane.

Symptoms

The onset may be acute or gradual, and the episodic symptoms are variable in their impact on different people and on one individual on different days; the course of the disease is unpredictable. The muscles of the eye, eyelids, tongue, jaw, and throat are the most commonly affected. Chewing and swallowing become increasingly difficult. The muscles of the extremities are also involved and in some cases, the respiratory muscles may also be affected. Fine motor skills (dexterity and manipulation) and gross motor skills (climbing stairs) are affected. Endurance is poor during the relapses. Loss of self-care skills and functional independence occur due to muscle weakness, range of motion, and reduced endurance. There is also a relative loss in leisure interests, social activities, and productivity.

Assessment Objectives

The OT will be responsible for assessing occupational performance areas and components. All areas assessed will be considered in relation to functional performance. Key areas for assessment include various performance areas and skills in order to identify realistic client-centered treatment goals.

Assessment of Performance Areas

- Activities of daily living: BADL and IADL skills
- Play and leisure skills
- Work/productivity skills
- Home management skills

Assessment of Performance Components

Sensory Processing
- Proprioceptive
- Tactile
- Vestibular
- Visual

Perceptual Processing
- Stereognosis
- Kinesthesia
- Position in space

Neuromusculoskeletal
- Range of motion
- Muscle tone
- Strength
- Endurance
- Postural control
- Postural alignment
- Soft tissue integrity

Motor
- Gross coordination
- Bilateral integration

- Motor control
- Praxis
- Fine coordination/dexterity
- Visual-motor integration
- Oral-motor control

Cognitive Integration

- Attention span
- Initiation of activity
- Problem solving
- Learning
- Generalization

Psychosocial Skills/Psychological Components

- Values
- Interests
- Self-concept
- Role performance
- Self-expression
- Time management

Standardized Assessment Tools

- ADL scales
- Occupational performance history
- Work history, job analysis review
- Leisure activities checklist
- Manual Muscle Test (withheld during acute stages of recovery)
- Range of Motion test
- Sensory testing
- Home evaluation for modification and assistive device/equipment recommendation

Standardized Tests

- Functional Independence Measure (FIM^{SM})
- Barthel Index
- Modified Interest Checklist
- Occupational Performance History Interview
- Jebson Hand function test

Prognosis and Outcome

The prognosis is generally good in mild cases of myasthenia gravis when regular medication is adequate to restore the patient's condition to near normal. Regular antibody-free plasma exchange (plasmapheresis), anticholinesterase drugs, glucocorticoids, corticosteroids and other immunosuppressive pharmacological agents, and thymectomy (removal of the thymus gland) are some of the other options that may be used in the management of myasthenia gravis. The primary desired outcome is improving or maintaining muscle strength, endurance, range of motion, ADL skills, and work and leisure skills. Assistive devices or environmental modifications may be necessary to optimize functional independence. Training family members in appropriate assistance of the client may be necessary. In a minority of cases, significant weakness and subsequent paralysis of the throat and respiratory failure may cause death.

osteoarthritis

Osteoarthritis (OA) is a progressive disorder characterized by altered hyaline cartilage, loss of articular cartilage, and hypertrophy of bone, producing osteophytes. Osteoarthritis is the most common articular disorder. It may be called degenerative joint disease or hypertrophic osteoarthritis (Beers & Berkow, 1999).

Etiology

Osteoarthritis (OA) is the most common rheumatic disease, affecting both men and women equally during middle age and beyond (ages 45–90), with its prevalence increasing with age. The progression of OA involves a two-stage process. First, a wearing down or deterioration of the articular cartilage occurs; next the build-up of bone around the margin of the joint creates the lumpy, enlarged appearance.

Symptoms

The stages of OA are frequently painless, with stiffness and limited range of motion as the primary presenting problems. There may be accompanying inflammation with pain and swelling of the affected joints in some cases. Common joints affected by OA include: hands, spine, knees, hips, and the metatarsal phalangeal joint of the great toe.

Assessment Objectives

The OT will be responsible for assessing occupational performance areas and components. All areas assessed will be considered in relation to functional performance. Key areas for assessment include various performance areas and skills in order to identify realistic client-centered treatment goals.

Assessment of Performance Areas

- Activities of daily living: BADL and IADL skills
- Home management: safety and adaptations
- Work/productivity
- Social/emotional
- Leisure activities

Assessment of Performance Components

Neuromusculoskeletal

- Range of motion
- Strength
- Endurance
- Postural control
- Postural alignment

Motor

- Gross coordination
- Fine coordination
- Dexterity

Cognitive Integration and Cognitive Components

- Learning
- Generalization

Psychosocial Skills

- Interests
- Self-concept
- Self-expression
- Coping

Standardized Assessment Tools

- Functional Independence Measure (FIM^{SM})
- Assessment of Motor and Process Skills (AMPS)
- Barthel Index
- Katz Index of ADL
- Klein-Bell Activities of Daily Living Scale
- Berg Balance Test
- Crawford Small Parts Dexterity Test
- Jebsen Hand Function Test
- Minnesota Rate of Manipulation Test (MRMT)
- Minnesota Manual Dexterity Test (MMDT)

- Purdue Pegboard
- Range of Motion (AROM/PROM)
- Muscle Test (MMT)
- Sensory Testing
- Tinetti Test of Balance and Gait
- Rhomberg Test of Balance
- Verbal Rating Scale
- Numeric Rating Scale
- Self-Esteem Scale
- Tennessee Self-Concept Scale—Revised (TSCS)
- Activity Index
- Interest Checklist
- Leisure Activities Bank
- Self-Assessment of Leisure Interests
- Goniometer
- Dynamometer
- Pinch meter

Prognosis and Outcome

Osteoarthritis is a slowly progressive disease. Management depends upon the client's ability and willingness to avoid or eliminate those activities and situations that may accelerate or aggravate the condition. Learning to adapt one's lifestyle and to live within the limitations of the disorder are positive strategies.

The desired outcome is to maintain and maximize ADL performance as long as possible with assistive devices and lifestyle adaptations. Pain management and energy conservation training may enhance occupational performance significantly.

osteoporosis

Osteoporosis is defined as low bone mass resulting from an excess of bone resorption over bone formation, with resultant bone fragility and increased risk of fracture.

Etiology

Caucasian females 50 years or older who are postmenopausal with inadequate dietary calcium intake, small bone structure, and who lead a sedentary lifestyle are most frequently affected. More than 50% of these women will develop an osteoporosis-related fracture during their remaining lifetime.

Symptoms

Most organ systems undergo degenerative change with aging. This can impede an older person's ability to safely interact with his or her environment. Examples of sensorimotor components that may be compromised are balance, visual acuity, focus, and resistance to glare. Neuromusculoskeletal components include decreased strength, endurance, and postural instability. Decline in motor functioning includes impaired motor control due to stiffened joints, decreased return of equilibrium after exertion, and decreased speed of response (Davis & Kirkland, 1988). Significant morbidity, mortality, and medical expense result from osteoporosis-related fractures. Spinal fractures, which occur in 25% of white women by age 65 years, cause pain, deformity, and disability. Hip fractures result in at least short-term institutionalization in more than 50% of patients and are associated with a mortality rate of 5-20% within the first year of fracture. It is estimated that more than 10% of women who sustain hip fractures become dependent in functional status, while many others never regain their full pre-fracture level of functional activity (Cummings, Kelsey, Nevitt, & O'Dowd, 1985).

Assessment Objectives

The OT will be responsible for assessing occupational performance areas and components. All areas assessed will be considered in relation to functional performance. Key areas for assessment include various performance areas and skills in order to identify realistic client-centered treatment goals.

Assessment of Performance Areas

- Activities of daily living: BADL and IADL skills
- Work/productivity skills
- Home management
- Play/leisure

Assessment of Performance Components

Sensory Processing
- Tactile
- Visual

Perceptual Processing
- Depth perception
- Spatial relations
- Topographical orientation

Neuromusculoskeletal
- Range of motion
- Strength
- Endurance
- Postural control
- Postural alignment

Motor
- Gross coordination
- Motor control
- Fine coordination/dexterity

Cognitive Integration and Cognitive Components
- Spatial operations
- Learning
- Generalization

Psychosocial Skills and Psychological Components
- Interests
- Role performance
- Time management
- Self-control

Standardized Assessment Tools

- Functional Independence Measure (FIM^{SM})
- Assessment of Motor and Process Skills (AMPS)
- Barthel Index
- Katz Index of ADL
- Klein-Bell Activities of Daily Living Scale
- Berg Balance Test
- Minnesota Manual Dexterity Test (MMDT)
- Purdue Pegboard
- Range of Motion (AROM/PROM)
- Muscle Test (MMT)
- Sensory Testing
- Tinetti Test of Balance and Gait
- Rhomberg Test of Balance
- Verbal Rating Scale
- Numeric Rating Scale
- Tennessee Self-Concept Scale—Revised (TSCS)
- Activity Index
- Interest Checklist
- Leisure Activities Bank

- Self-Assessment of Leisure Interests
- Goniometer
- Dynamometer
- Pinch meter

Prognosis and Outcome

Osteoporosis is a common bone disorder, particularly of older women, with significant morbidity and mortality resulting from spinal deformity and hip fractures. Preventive strategies include adequate lifetime calcium intake, weight-bearing exercise, and postmenopausal hormone replacement. Treatment for osteoporosis is less well established, with each therapy posing potential barriers including cost, side effects, and lack of long-term efficacy.

paraplegia See spinal cord injury.

Parkinson's disease

Parkinson's disease is a slowly progressive degenerative disorder of the basal ganglia in the central nervous system. The disease is characterized by slow and decreased movement (bradykinesia), muscular rigidity, resting tremor, and postural instability (Beers & Berkow, 1999).

Etiology

The cause of Parkinson's disease is not known. Parkinson's disease may be a disease of multiple causes. Infectious, genetic, and immunologic causes are considerations, as are arteriosclerosis, encephalitis, anoxia, and trauma.

Symptoms

May not be readily apparent in a newly diagnosed and medically well-managed case. As the disease progresses and as the client ages, continuous medication management may lead to side effects, including: drug-related dystonia, muscle contractions, repetitive movements, abnormal postures, and sudden, non-purposeful movements.

Assessment Objectives

The OT is responsible for reviewing the available medical record, obtaining a brief functional history, and assessing occupational performance areas and components. All areas assessed will be considered in relation to functional performance. Key areas for assessment include various performance areas and skills in order to identify realistic client-centered treatment goals.

Assessment of Performance Areas

- Activities of daily living: BADL and IADL skills
- Work and productive skills: home management, and home safety
- Vocational activities: Retirement planning
- Leisure activities: Leisure exploration and performance

Assessment of Performance Components

Sensory Processing
- Tactile
- Proprioceptive
- Vestibular
- Visual

Perceptual Processing
- Stereognosis
- Kinesthesia
- Body scheme
- Position in space
- Depth perception
- Spatial relations
- Topographical orientation

Neuromusculoskeletal
- Range of motion
- Muscle tone
- Strength
- Endurance
- Postural control
- Postural alignment
- Soft tissue integrity

Motor
- Gross coordination
- Bilateral integration
- Motor control
- Praxis
- Fine coordination/dexterity
- Visual-motor integration
- Oral-motor control

Cognitive Integration and Cognitive Components
- Level of arousal
- Orientation
- Attention span
- Recognition
- Initiation of activity
- Termination of activity
- Memory and sequencing
- Spatial operations
- Problem solving
- Learning
- Generalization

Psychosocial Skills
- Interests
- Role performance
- Self-expression
- Coping skills
- Time management

Standardized Assessment Tools
- Functional Independence Measure (FIM^{SM})
- Assessment of Motor and Process Skills (AMPS)
- Klein-Bell Activities of Daily Living Scale
- Kohlman Evaluation of Living Skills (KELS)
- Range of Motion (ROM)
- Muscle Test (MMT)
- Tinetti Balance Test
- Minnesota Rate of Manipulation
- Purdue Peg Board
- Global Deterioration Scale (GDS)
- Blessed Dementia Rating Scale
- Cognitive Assessment of Minnesota (CAM)
- The Middlesex Elderly Assessment of Mental State (MEAMS)
- Mini-Mental State Exam (MMSE)
- Clinic-based and road-based driving assessments
- Yesavage Geriatric Depression Screen

Prognosis and Outcome

Parkinson's disease is a progressive, degenerative disorder. Occupational therapy assessment and treatment intervention may slow the extent of disability and enhance functional performance, though it will not affect the course of the disease. The desired outcome is to maximize and maintain one's ability to perform relevant activities of daily living. Incorporation of adaptive skills and assistive devices and technology into one's lifestyle can assist in facilitating positive functional performance of daily life skills.

personality disorders

Personality disorders are pervasive, inflexible, and stable personality traits that deviate from cultural norms and cause distress or functional impairment (American Psychiatric Association, 1994). Having a personality disorder can negatively affect one's work, family, and social life. Personality disorders exist on a continuum so they can be mild to more severe in terms of how pervasive they are and to what extent an individual exhibits the features of a particular personality disorder. While most people can live relatively normal lives with mild personality disorders (personality traits), during times of increased stress or external pressures (work, family, a new relationship, etc.), the symptoms of the personality disorder will gain strength and begin to seriously interfere with emotional and psychological functioning.

There are ten different types of personality disorders that can be grouped into three major clusters according to the *DSM-IV* (American Psychiatric Association, 1994), which all have various emphases:

Odd and Eccentric Personality Disorders
- Paranoid Personality Disorder (suspicious, distrustful)
- Schizoid Personality Disorder (socially distant, detached)
- Schizotypal Personality Disorder (odd, eccentric)

Dramatic, Emotional, or Erratic Personality Disorders
- Antisocial Personality Disorder (impulsive, aggressive, manipulative)
- Borderline Personality Disorder (impulsive, self-destructive, unstable)
- Histrionic Personality Disorder (emotional, dramatic, theatrical)
- Narcissistic Personality Disorder (boastful, egotistical, "superiority complex")

Anxious or Fearful Personality Disorders
- Avoidant Personality Disorder (passive, anxious)
- Dependent Personality Disorder (dependent, submissive, clinging)
- Obsessive-Compulsive Personality Disorder (perfectionist, rigid, controlling)

Etiology

Personality disorders may be caused by a combination of parental upbringing, latent or natural personality, and social development associated with early childhood experiences, as well as genetic and biological factors. Research has not narrowed down the cause to any factor at this time. These disorders will most often manifest themselves during increased times of stress and interpersonal difficulties in one's life. Therefore, treatment most often focuses on increasing one's coping mechanisms and interpersonal skills.

Symptoms

People with a personality disorder possess several distinct psychological problems that include: disturbances in self-image, inability to have successful interpersonal relationships, inappropriate range of emotions, difficulty distinguishing their own needs from others' needs, and poor impulse control. These disturbances come together to create a pervasive pattern of behavior and inner experience that is quite different from the norms of the individual's culture. These disturbances often tend to be expressed in behaviors that appear more dramatic than what society considers usual and is manifested in at least two of the following areas: affectivity, cognition, impulse control, and interpersonal functioning.

Assessment Objectives

The OT will be responsible for assessing occupational performance areas and components. All areas assessed will be considered in relation to functional performance. Key areas for assessment include various performance areas and skills in order to identify realistic client-centered treatment goals.

Assessment of Performance Areas

- Activities of daily living: BADL and IADL skills
- Play and leisure skills

- School/educational setting if applicable
- Work/productivity skills

Assessment of Performance Components

Cognitive Integration

- Level of arousal
- Orientation
- Attention span
- Problem solving
- Learning
- Generalization

Psychosocial Skills/Psychological Components

- Values
- Interests
- Self-concept
- Social conduct
- Role performance
- Interpersonal skills
- Self-control
- Self-expression
- Time management

Standardized Assessment Tools

- ADL scales
- Occupational performance history
- Work history, job analysis review
- Leisure activities checklist
- Cognitive scales
- Perception evaluation scales

Standardized Tests

- Allen Cognitive Level Test
- Allen Diagnostic Module
- Assessment of Motor and Process Skills, 2nd ed. (AMPS)
- Kohlman Evaluation of Living Skills
- Mini Mental State Examination
- Modified Interest Checklist
- Occupational Performance History Interview
- Self-Esteem Scale
- Worker Role Inventory

Prognosis and Outcome

Prognosis cannot be generalized as good. People with personality disorders usually require long-term therapy to make modest gains. Drugs have limited effects and can be misused or used in suicide attempts. When anxiety and depression result from a personality disorder, drugs are only moderately effective. For a person with personality disorders, anxiety and depression may have a positive significance, experiencing unwanted consequences of his or her disorder or undertaking some needed self-examination. Because personality disorders are particularly difficult to treat, the OT's experience, enthusiasm, and an understanding of the patient's expected areas of emotional sensitivity and usual ways of coping are important. Kindness and direction alone do not change personality disorders. Family members can act in ways that either reinforce or diminish the patient's problematic behavior or thoughts, so their involvement is helpful and often essential.

postpolio syndrome, postpoliomyelitis syndrome

Postpolio syndrome occurs in individuals who have been affected by paralytic poliomyelitis. It is characterized by pain, reduced endurance, muscle fatigue and weakness, fasciculations, and atrophy that occurs years after the initial diagnosis of paralytic poliomyelitis (Beers & Berkow, 1999). The number of postpolio cases is reducing considerably in the United States. However, poliomyelitis and postpolio syndrome are fairly common in some Asian and African countries.

Etiology

It occurs in persons with a history of poliomyelitis. The exact cause is unknown. It is proposed that it may be due to the loss of anterior horn cells in the spinal cord as a natural aging process complicated by initial cell loss as a result of polio (Beers & Berkow, 1999). Another explanation is that the weakness is superimposed by conditions such as degenerative joint disease and related weakness to muscles and ligaments, disk herniation, diabetes mellitus, muscle overuse, compressive neuropathy, or myofascial pain.

Symptoms

Symptoms include muscle pain, muscle fatigue and weakness, decreased endurance, fasciculations, and atrophy of affected muscles.

Assessment Objectives

The OT will be responsible for assessing occupational perform-ance areas and components. The OT will be involved in assess-ment and management throughout the course of the patient's stay in the acute and rehabilitation setting. All areas assessed will be considered in relation to functional performance. Key areas for assessment include various performance areas and skills in order to identify realistic client-centered treatment goals.

Assessment of Performance Areas

- Activities of daily living: BADL and IADL skills
- Play and leisure skills
- Work/productivity skills

Assessment of Performance Components

Sensory Processing
- Proprioceptive
- Tactile

Perceptual Processing
- Kinesthesia
- Position in space
- Body scheme

Neuromusculoskeletal
- Range of motion
- Muscle tone
- Strength
- Endurance
- Postural control
- Postural alignment
- Soft tissue integrity

Motor
- Gross coordination
- Bilateral integration
- Motor control
- Praxis

- Fine coordination/dexterity
- Laterality
- Oral-motor control

Cognitive Integration
- Level of arousal
- Problem solving
- Learning
- Generalization

Psychosocial Skills/Psychological Components
- Interests
- Self-concept
- Role performance
- Interpersonal skills
- Self-expression
- Time management

Standardized Assessment Tools

- ADL scales
- Manual Muscle Test
- Range of Motion Test
- Sensory testing
- Evaluation of physical environments such as home and workplace
- Evaluation of assistive devices used
- Work history and job analysis
- Leisure activities checklist
- Endurance testing

Standardized Tests
- Functional Independence Measure (FIM[SM])
- Barthel Index
- Klein-Bell Activities of Daily Living Scale
- Kohlman Evaluation of Living Skills
- Modified Interest Checklist
- Occupational Performance History Interview

Prognosis and Outcome

Prognosis depends on the amount of muscle involvement and muscle weakness. Individuals may be able to gain functional independence in many of their daily tasks with the use of adaptive devices or adaptation to their physical environment. Time management and work simplification tasks may be needed to improve or maintain functional independence.

post traumatic stress disorder

Also known as shell shock or battle fatigue syndrome, post traumatic stress disorder (PTSD) is an anxiety disorder that features the development of characteristic symptoms following exposure to an extreme traumatic stressor involving direct personal experience of an event (American Psychiatric Association, 1994). Extreme trauma is a terrifying event that a person has experienced, witnessed, or learned about, especially one that is life threatening or causes physical harm. It can be a single event or a repeated experience. The stress caused by the trauma can affect all aspects of a person's life including mental, emotional, and physical well-being. Seventy percent of adults in the United States have experienced a traumatic event at least once in their lives, and up to 20% go on to develop PTSD (Post Traumatic Stress Disorder Alliance). About 3.6% of U.S. adults ages 18–54 (5.2 million people) have PTSD during the course of a given year (National Institute of Mental Health, 2001). The most common precipitating events for PTSD in women were rape and physical assault (33.8% and 32.3% of reported events, respectively). For men, seeing someone seriously hurt or killed and physical assault were the most prevalent (25.3% and 20.3%). Women and men were equally likely to have been exposed to trauma (Friedman, 2001).

Signs and symptoms of PTSD typically appear within 3 months of the traumatic event. But in some instances, they may not occur until years after the event. Everyone who experiences trauma does not require treatment; some recover with the help of family, friends, or clergy. But many do need professional treatment to recover from the psychological damage that can result from experiencing, witnessing, or participating in an overwhelmingly traumatic event.

Other factors that may increase the likelihood of developing post traumatic stress disorder (Mayo Clinic, 2001) include:

- Previous history of depression or other emotional disorder
- Previous history of physical or sexual abuse
- Family history of anxiety
- Early separation from parents

- Being part of a dysfunctional family
- Alcohol abuse
- Drug abuse

Etiology

PTSD occurs in response to situations or events such as natural or man-made disasters, physical or sexual abuse, violent crime or accident, or acts of war.

Symptoms

PTSD usually appears within 3 months of the trauma, but sometimes the disorder appears later. PTSD's symptoms fall into three categories:

Intrusion

Memories of the trauma reoccur unexpectedly, and episodes called "flashbacks" intrude into their current lives. Flashback happens in nightmares or in sudden, vivid memories with painful emotions and may be so strong that individuals almost feel like they are actually experiencing the trauma again or seeing it unfold before their eyes.

Avoidance

Avoidance symptoms affect relationships with others. The person often avoids close emotional ties with family, colleagues, and friends. The person with PTSD avoids situations or activities that are reminders of the original traumatic event because such exposure may cause symptoms to worsen.

Hyperarousal

Hyperarousal PTSD can cause those who have it to act as if they are constantly threatened by the trauma that caused their illness. They can become suddenly irritable or explosive, even when they are not provoked. They may have trouble concentrating or remembering current information, and because of their terrifying nightmares, they may develop insomnia.

Assessment Objectives

The OT will be responsible for assessing occupational performance areas and components. All areas assessed will be considered in relation to functional performance. Key areas for assessment include various performance areas and skills in order to identify realistic client-centered treatment goals.

Assessment of Performance Areas

- Activities of daily living: BADL and IADL skills
- Home management skills
- Play and leisure skills
- School/educational setting if applicable
- Work/productivity skills

Assessment of Performance Components

Sensory Processing
- Visual
- Auditory

Perceptual Processing
- Body scheme

Cognitive Integration
- Level of arousal
- Orientation
- Recognition
- Attention span
- Memory
- Sequencing
- Categorization
- Initiation of activity
- Termination of activity
- Concept formation
- Spatial operations
- Problem solving
- Learning
- Generalization

Psychosocial Skills/Psychological Components
- Values
- Interests
- Self-concept
- Social conduct
- Role performance
- Interpersonal skills
- Self-control
- Self-expression
- Time management

Standardized Assessment Tools

- ADL scales
- Occupational performance history
- Work history, job analysis review
- Leisure activities checklist
- Cognitive scales
- Perception evaluation scales

Standardized Tests

- Assessment of Motor and Process Skills, 2nd ed.
- Mini Mental State Examination
- Modified Interest Checklist
- Occupational Performance History Interview
- Self-Esteem Scale
- Worker Role Inventory
- Canadian Occupational Performance Measure (COPM)
- Kohlman Evaluation of Living Skills
- Barth Time Construction
- Social Readjustment Rating Scale

Prognosis and Outcome

The symptoms of PTSD disappear with time in some cases, whereas in others they persist for many years. PTSD often occurs with—or leads to—other psychiatric illnesses, such as depression. Having post traumatic stress disorder may place an individual at a higher risk for depression (which shares many of the same symptoms as post traumatic stress disorder), drug abuse, alcohol abuse, eating disorders, and divorce. Stress management training, cognitive-behavioral therapy, group therapy, and desensitization-exposure therapy along with pharmacotherapy (used to relieve the most distressing symptoms) have good outcomes in people with PTSD. Patient education and family education are very important.

prenatal exposure to cocaine

Cocaine is considered one of the most dangerous illicit drugs available today. Recent epidemiological data indicate that cocaine use is widespread in society. The National Institute on Drug Abuse (NIDA) estimated that 5 million Americans are regular users of cocaine, 20 to 30 million other Americans have tried the drug on at least one occasion, and 5,000 additional individuals try cocaine for the first time each day. In addition to effects on physical development, neurological and behavioral abnormalities observed in cocaine-exposed human infants have included poor performance on the Brazelton Neonatal Behavioral Assessment Scale (BNBAS), tremulousness, and muscle rigidity.

Etiology

Cocaine is a central nervous system (CNS) stimulant, demonstrating both anesthetic and vasoconstrictive effects. Cocaine will travel into the placenta where it is assumed to cause significant vasoconstriction, diminished blood flow to the fetus, and resultant periods of hypoxia. The effect that this drug has on the developing fetus is probably a function of the stage of fetal development as well as the degree and extent of the drug exposure itself. It is significant to note that cocaine is an appetite depressant, and that the mother may not be adequately nourished, leading to low birth weight and small head circumference babies at delivery.

Symptoms

Clinical data indicate that the neonate exposed *in utero* to cocaine may have a lower gestational age at delivery, lower birth weight, and decreased body length and head circumference. Studies have also reported associations between cocaine use during pregnancy and the occurrence of fetal anomalies, including an increase in skull malformations such as parietal bone defects, exencephaly, and interparietal encephalocele, limb defects, urogenital system anomalies such as "prune belly syndrome," and neural tube defects. Intrauterine fetal death also occurs more frequently in pregnant cocaine users than in nonusers. Several studies have reported an increased incidence of sudden infant death syndrome (SIDS) with cocaine use (Zuckerman, 1996). Many cocaine-exposed human neonates show evidence of physical and/or behavioral abnormalities that may be due, at least in part, to cocaine exposure. Other factors that affect physical and behavioral development are seen frequently in cocaine-abusing mothers, and the potentially confounding effects of these variables cannot be ignored. *In utero* exposure to cocaine produces:

- Neonatal withdrawal (may persist for several days to several weeks)
- Tremulousness

- Irritability
- Abnormal sleep patterns
- Poor feeding
- High-pitched cry
- Muscle rigidity
- Jitteriness
- Hypertonicity
- Vomiting
- Diarrhea
- Diaphoresis
- Convulsions
- Hyperventilation

Assessment Objectives

The OT will be responsible for assessing occupational performance areas and components. All areas assessed will be considered in relation to functional performance. Key areas for assessment include various performance areas and skills in order to identify realistic client-centered treatment goals.

Assessment of Performance Areas

- Activities of daily living: BADL skills
- Social/emotional performance
- Play and leisure skills
- School/educational skills and environment
- Neurodevelopmental
- Physical development
- Sensory processing
- Neurobehavioral status
- Psychosocial/physical environment

Assessment of Performance Components

Sensory Processing

- Tactile
- Proprioceptive
- Vestibular
- Visual
- Auditory
- Olfactory
- Gustatory

Perceptual Processing
- Kinesthesia
- Pain response
- Visual closure
- Figure ground
- Spatial relations
- Topographical orientation

Neuromusculoskeletal
- Reflex
- Range of motion
- Muscle tone
- Strength
- Endurance
- Postural control
- Postural alignment

Motor
- Gross coordination
- Crossing the midline
- Bilateral integration
- Motor control
- Praxis
- Fine coordination/dexterity
- Visual-motor integration
- Oral-motor control

Cognitive Integration and Cognitive Components
- Level of arousal
- Recognition
- Attention span
- Initiation of activity
- Learning
- Generalization

Psychosocial Skills
- Social conduct
- Self-expression
- Coping
- Self-control
- Role performance

Standardized Assessment Tools

- Miller Assessment for Preschoolers (MAP)
- Bayley Scales of Infant Development-II (BSID-II)
- Movement Assessment of Infants (MAI)
- Peabody Developmental Motor Scales (PDMS)
- Fagan Test of Infant Intelligence (FTII)
- Test of Sensory Functions in Infants (TSFI)
- DeGangi-Berk Test of Sensory Integration (DBTSI)
- Developmental Hand Dysfunction: Theory, Assessment, and Treatment
- Parenting Stress Index-Short Form
- Early Coping Inventory (ECI)
- Child Abuse Potential Inventory (CAPI), 2nd ed.
- Child Behavior Checklist for Ages 2–3
- Toddler and Infant Motor Evaluation (TIME)
- Observation Scale for Mother-Infant Interaction During Feeding
- School Assessment of Motor and Process Skills (SAMPS)
- Wee Functional Independence Measure (Wee FIM^{SM})

Prognosis and Outcome

Maternal cocaine use has been clearly associated with intrauterine growth retardation, particularly low birth weight and microcephaly, in human studies. Transient neonatal withdrawal has also been associated with *in utero* exposure to cocaine. Other possible associations include spontaneous abortions, malformations, and SIDS. Although these risks are biologically plausible, further studies are needed to assess the long-term neurobehavioral effects of cocaine use during pregnancy.

rheumatoid arthritis

Rheumatoid arthritis (RA) is a chronic condition that is characterized by inflammation of peripheral joints, resulting in progressive destruction of the articular and periarticular structures (Beers & Berkow, 1999). According to the Arthritis Foundation (2001), there are seven classifications of RA:

- Morning stiffness: morning stiffness in and around the joints
- Arthritis of 3 or more joints: soft tissue swelling of 3 or more joints

- Arthritis of hand joints: at least one area swollen in the hand (wrist, PIPs, MCPs, and MTPs are involved)
- Symmetric arthritis: simultaneous involvement of the same joints on both sides of the body (mostly hand joints)
- Rheumatoid nodules: subcutaneous nodules over bony prominences, extensor surfaces, or in juxta-articular regions
- Serum rheumatoid factor: abnormal amounts of serum rheumatoid factor
- Radiographic changes: radiographs showing erosions or unequivocal decalcification

Etiology

Rheumatoid arthritis is more prevalent in women than men. Definite cause is unknown. Possible causes include autoimmune deficiency, environmental factors, and genetic predisposition.

Symptoms

Rheumatoid arthritis leads to inflammation of synovial joints. The disease ranges from mild to severe leading to permanent joint damage. The joints become painful, stiff, and hot. Range of motion (ROM) is limited because of pain and edema. Muscle weakness might result from disuse. Morning stiffness is a common sign of RA. The course of the disease is characterized by exacerbations and remissions. The person's level of function varies from independence in ADLs to complete dependence as a result of joint pain and ROM limitations. Lack of motivation and depression might result due to inability to perform daily activities.

Assessment Objectives

The OT will be responsible for assessing occupational performance areas and components. All areas assessed will be considered in relation to functional performance. Key areas for assessment include various performance areas and skills in order to identify realistic client-centered treatment goals.

Assessment of Performance Areas

- Activities of daily living: BADL and IADL skills
- Home management skills
- Vocational/avocational performance
- Play and leisure skills
- Work/productivity skills

Assessment of Performance Components

Sensory Processing
- Proprioceptive
- Tactile

Perceptual Processing
- Stereognosis
- Kinesthesia
- Position in space
- Body scheme

Neuromusculoskeletal
- Range of motion
- Strength
- Endurance
- Postural control
- Postural alignment

Motor
- Gross coordination
- Bilateral integration
- Fine coordination/dexterity

Cognitive Integration
- Attention span
- Memory
- Problem solving
- Learning
- Generalization

Psychosocial Skills/Psychological Components
- Interests
- Self-concept
- Social conduct
- Role performance
- Self-expression
- Time management

Standardized Assessment Tools

- Manual muscle test
- Goniometer
- Dynamometer
- Pinch meter
- Hand function tests

- Sensory testing
- ADL scales
- Home evaluation
- Assistive devices to evaluate ADL, work, and leisure skills
- Occupational performance history
- Leisure activities checklist

Standardized Tests
- Functional Independence Measure (FIM^SM)
- Barthel Index
- Modified Interest Checklist
- Occupational Performance History Interview
- Jebson Hand Function Test
- Worker Role Inventory
- Stanford Health Assessment Questionnaire

Prognosis and Outcome

Prognosis varies depending on the severity of the condition and the amount of joint involvement. Joint range, muscle strength, and daily function can be maintained or increased with medication, exercise, splinting, adaptive equipment, home modifications, and energy conservation techniques. The person may be able to maintain a productive life within the limits of one's disability. Family counseling and psychological help may be needed if the person suffers from depression and adjustment to the condition.

schizophrenia

Schizophrenia is considered a group of related psychotic disorders, rather than a single diagnostic entity. Disturbances in thought processes and the psychotic symptoms associated with schizophrenia can lead to difficulties with a wide variety of life skills and performance components.

Etiology

Approximately 1% of the population of industrialized countries is diagnosed as schizophrenic. There are approximately 200,000 patients who are institutionalized in hospitals and nursing homes in the United States, and another 400,000 individuals with schizophrenia living in community-based settings including group, foster care, and private independent dwellings (NIMH, 1999). The age of onset is typically early adulthood, but schizophrenia can appear in adolescence. Schizophrenia is equally common in males and females. For the diagnosis to be made, the symptoms must be severe enough to impair social and occupational function and must be present for a minimum of six months (American Psychiatric Association, 1994).

Symptoms

Characteristic symptoms of schizophrenia include disturbances of:

- Thought content
- Process (form) of thought
- Perception
- Affect
- Volition
- Sense of self

There may also be social withdrawal and disturbed psychomotor behavior. No single feature is always present, though delusions, hallucinations, and disorganized speech and behavior are commonly demonstrated in schizophrenia.

Assessment Objectives

The OT will be responsible for assessing occupational performance areas and components. All areas assessed will be considered in relation to functional performance. Key areas for assessment include various performance areas and skills in order to identify realistic client-centered treatment goals.

Assessment of Performance Areas

- Activities of daily living: BADLs and simple IADLs
- Work and productivity activities
- Prevocational and vocational performance
- Play/leisure activities

Assessment of Performance Components

Cognitive Integration and Cognitive Components

- Level of arousal
- Orientation
- Recognition
- Attention span
- Initiation of activity
- Termination of activity
- Memory

- Sequencing
- Categorization
- Concept formation
- Spatial operations
- Problem solving
- Learning
- Generalization

Psychosocial Skills and Psychological Component

- Values
- Interests
- Self-concept
- Role performance
- Social conduct
- Interpersonal skills
- Self-expression
- Coping skills
- Time management
- Self-control

Standardized Assessment Tools

- Allen Cognitive Levels
- Assessment of Motor and Process Skills (AMPS)
- Assessment of Communication and Interactional Skills (ACIS)
- Canadian Occupational Performance Measure (COPM)
- Cognitive Adaptive Skills Evaluation (CASE)
- Functional Assessment Scale (FAS)
- Geriatric Depression Scale (GDS)
- Geriatric Rating Scale (GRS)
- Kohlman Evaluation of Living Skills (KELS)
- Milwaukee Evaluation of Daily Living Skills (MEDLS)
- NPI Interest Checklist
- Role Checklist
- Street Survival Skills Questionnaire (SSSQ)
- Stress Management Questionnaire (SMQ)

Prognosis and Outcome

The course of schizophrenia and the prognosis is highly variable. Some of the contributing factors include: the person's symptoms, the sub-type of schizophrenia, acceptance of treatment approaches, and acceptance and utilization of treatment medications. According to Stevens (1997), one of three possible courses of the illness may be experienced:

• A single episode of symptoms with almost total recovery
• Repeated episodes with moderate recovery in between
• A progressive slide into long-term disability

When compared with other patients with psychosis, persons with schizophrenia recover more slowly and are less likely to show improvement in follow-up periods. Individuals with schizophrenia show a poorer outcome than those with other psychoses, such as mood disorders (Harrow, Sands, Silverstein, & Goldberg, 1997).

sensory integrative dysfunction

Sensory integration is the critical function of the brain that is responsible for producing a composite picture of an individual and the environment. It is the organization of sensory information for ongoing use. Sensory experiences include touch, movement, body awareness, sight, sound, and the pull of gravity. Sensory integration is the ability to synthesize, organize, and process sensory information received from the body and the environment to produce purposeful goal-directed responses (Arkwright, 1998). Sensory integration provides a crucial foundation for later, more complex learning and behavior.

For most children, sensory integration develops in the course of ordinary childhood activities. Motor planning ability is a natural outcome of the process, as is the ability to adapt to incoming sensations. But for some children, sensory integration does not develop as efficiently as it should. When the process is disordered, a number of problems in learning, development, or behavior may become evident.

Sensory integrative dysfunction is a developmental disorder resulting from difficulty with processing sensory input. Sensory integrative dysfunction can broadly be classified as sensory modulation disorders, adaptive movement response disorders, and sensory discrimination and perceptual disorders. Tactile defensiveness, gravitational insecurity, hyporesponsivity, vestibular processing disorder, developmental dyspraxia, tactile discrimination, proprioceptive perception, and visual perception are some of the common conditions of sensory integrative dysfunction.

Sensory integration theory is based in neuroscience and was formulated by Jean Ayres (1972) to describe behavior in children with learning disabilities. The basic concept of sensory integration is that the central nervous system receives, filters, organizes, and integrates stimuli in order for an individual to make an adaptive response. This concept is used to explain behavior across ages and relates to many diagnostic groups.

Research clearly identifies sensory integrative problems in children with developmental or learning difficulties. Independent studies show that a sensory integrative dysfunction can be found in up to 70% of children who are considered learning disabled by schools. Sensory integrative problems are not confined to children with learning disabilities. They transect all age groups as well as all intellectual levels and social strata (South Shore Educational Collaborative).

Etiology

The cause of sensory integrative dysfunction is unknown, though the origin is assumed to be within the processing centers of the central nervous system.

Symptoms

The following are some of the most common symptoms of sensory integrative dysfunction:

- Hypersensitivity to touch, movement, smells, sights, or sounds
- Hyporeactive to sensory stimulation
- Postural control issues
- Poor attention and concentration
- Activity level that is unusually high or low
- Coordination problems
- Delays in speech, language, motor skills, or academic achievement
- Poor organization
- Impulsive; lacking in self-control
- Poor self-concept, self-esteem
- Poor social interactions and emotional adjustments

Assessment Objectives

Occupational therapy for children with sensory integration dysfunction enhances their ability to process lower level senses related to alertness, understanding movement, body position, and touch. The OT will be responsible for assessing occupational performance areas and components. All areas assessed will be considered in relation to functional performance. Key areas for assessment include various performance areas and skills in order to identify realistic client-centered treatment goals.

Assessment of Performance Areas

- Activities of daily living: BADL and simple IADL skills
- Play and leisure skills
- School/educational setting if applicable

Assessment of Performance Components

Sensory Processing
- Proprioceptive
- Tactile
- Vestibular
- Visual
- Auditory
- Gustatory
- Olfactory

Perceptual Processing
- Kinesthesia
- Position in space
- Right-left discrimination
- Body scheme
- Depth perception
- Spatial relations
- Topographical orientation

Neuromusculoskeletal
- Muscle tone
- Endurance
- Postural control
- Postural alignment

Motor
- Gross coordination
- Bilateral integration
- Motor control
- Praxis
- Fine coordination/dexterity

- Laterality
- Crossing the midline
- Visual-motor integration
- Oral-motor control

Cognitive Integration

- Level of arousal
- Attention span
- Initiation of activity
- Termination of activity
- Concept formation
- Spatial operations
- Problem solving
- Learning
- Generalization

Psychosocial Skills/Psychological Components

- Interests
- Self-concept
- Social conduct
- Role performance
- Interpersonal skills
- Self-control
- Self-expression

Standardized Assessment Tools

- ADL scales
- Developmental scales
- Hand function tests
- Play scales
- Prevocational skill testing for adults and young adults
- Cognitive and perceptual tests

Standardized Tests

- DeGangi-Berk Test of Sensory Integration (TSI)
- Assessment of Motor and Process Skills (AMPS), 2nd ed.
- Bayley Scales of Infant Development-II (BSID-II)
- Children's Playfulness Scale
- Developmental Test of Visual Perception, 2nd Edition (DTVP-2)
- Functional Independence Measure (FIM^SM) and Functional Independence Measure for Children (Wee FIM^SM)

- Klein-Bell Activities of Daily Living Scale
- Peabody Developmental Motor Scales (PDMS)
- Miller Assessment for Preschoolers (MAP)
- Play Observation
- Sensory Integration and Praxis Tests (SIPT)
- Sensory Profile
- Vineland Adaptive Behavior Scales-Revised (VABS-R)

Prognosis and Outcome

The prognosis and outcome in sensory integrative dysfunction is variable due to the variety of problems. Coexisting diagnoses may also limit the outcome of sensory integrative therapy.

shell shock See post traumatic stress disorder.

spina bifida

Spina bifida is defective closure of the vertebral column. It is one of the most serious neural tube defects compatible with prolonged life. Varieties include: the occult (closed) type with no neurological findings, to a completely open spine (rachischisis) with severe neurological impairment and multiple disabilities. Problems with closed defects include compression of the spinal cord and stretched spinal cord (tethered cord). In spina bifida cystica or operata (open), the protruding sac can contain meninges (meningocele), spinal cord (myelocele), or both (myelomeningocele).

Etiology

Failure of the neural tube to close properly during fetal development remains the elusive cause of spina bifida. Although the exact cause is unknown, lack of folic acid is suspected in about 50% of cases. Environmental and genetic components may also play a role. Spina bifida occurs during the first month of embryonic life, when the central nervous system is forming. If the developing tube fails to close, an opening occurs called a neural tube defect. Usually the defect occurs in the lumbar, low thoracic, or sacral region of the spine and extends three to six vertebral segments. The incidence of spina bifida is about 1:1,000 in the United States. It is the second most common birth defect after Down syndrome (Williamson, 1987). Boys are more frequently affected than girls (Reed, 2001).

Symptoms

When the spinal cord or lumbosacral nerve roots are involved, varying degrees of paralysis occur below the involved level. Since the paralysis occurs in the fetus, orthopedic problems can present at birth, such as hydrocephalus, clubfoot, arthrogryposis, or dislocated hip. The paralysis generally affects bladder and renal functions.

Assessment Objectives

The OT will assess the child with neural tube defects within the context of the various environments in which the child functions. The OT will be responsible for assessing occupational performance areas and components. All areas assessed will be considered in relation to functional performance. Key areas for assessment include various performance areas and skills in order to identify realistic client-centered treatment goals.

Assessment of Performance Areas

- Activities of daily living: BADL and simple IADL skills
- Work and productive areas: Educational, prevocational and vocational activities
- Play/leisure activities

Assessment of Performance Components

Sensory Processing
- Tactile
- Proprioceptive
- Vestibular
- Visual
- Auditory
- Olfactory

Perceptual Processing
- Stereognosis
- Kinesthesia
- Pain response
- Body scheme
- Right-left discrimination
- Form constancy
- Position in space
- Visual closure

- Figure ground
- Depth perception
- Spatial relations
- Topographical orientation

Neuromusculoskeletal
- Reflex
- Range of motion
- Muscle tone
- Strength
- Endurance
- Postural control
- Postural alignment
- Soft tissue integrity

Motor
- Gross coordination
- Crossing the midline
- Laterality
- Bilateral integration
- Motor control
- Praxis
- Fine coordination/dexterity
- Visual-motor integration
- Oral-motor control

Cognitive Integration and Cognitive Components
- Level of arousal
- Orientation
- Recognition
- Attention span
- Initiation of activity
- Termination of activity
- Memory
- Sequencing
- Spatial operations
- Problem solving
- Learning
- Generalization

Psychosocial Skills
- Interests
- Self-concept

- Social conduct
- Interpersonal skills
- Self-expression
- Coping
- Self-control

Standardized Assessment Tools

- Miller Assessment for Preschoolers (MAP)
- Movement Assessment for Infants (MAI)
- School Assessment of Motor and Process Skills (SAMPS)
- Toddler and Infant Motor Evaluation (TIME)
- The Beery-Buktenica Developmental Test of Visual-Motor Integration (VMI-4)
- Bruininks-Oseretsky Test of Motor Proficiency (BOTMP)
- Motor-Free Visual Perception Test-Revised (MVPT-R)
- Peabody Developmental Motor Scales (PDMS)
- Test of Visual-Motor Skills—Revised (TVMS-R)
- Test of Visual-Perceptual Skills—Revised (TVPS-R)
- Vineland Behavioral Scales (VBS)
- Wee Functional Independence Measure (WeeFIM^{SM})

Prognosis and Outcome

Though lower extremity impairment is expected in children with spina bifida, reduced control of upper limbs is also common. Hydrocephalus may cause damage to the motor cortex, affecting perceptual function as well. Deprivation or distortion of movement experiences interferes with efficiency of motor planning, which depends on the feedback and integration of sensory information from successful motor experiences. The child with spina bifida may have difficulty with cognitive performance components, such as the complex sequences required for eating, dressing, and handwriting (Williamson, 1987).

The neural tube damage caused by neural tube defects usually results in some sensory-processing deficits that affect the development of motor planning, visual-perceptual skills, and bilateral coordination. Additional sensory deficits are specific to sensory systems. An example being the visual system may be impaired with refractive errors or nystagmus.

Children with myelomeningocele and hydrocephalus score lower than normal children on tests of visual perception (Williamson,

1987). Exaggerated, emotional responses to specific sensory stimuli are caused by hyperresponsivity to sensory input eliciting primitive, protective responses. Auditory defensiveness has also been reported frequently in children with hydrocephalus.

Bowel and bladder control presents a special problem for the child with spina bifida, though as they grow older, most children can gradually become independent in bowel and bladder management (Williamson, 1987).

Approximately half of all children with myelomeningocele use a wheelchair, either as their primary means of mobility or for distance mobility. Power wheelchairs or scooters may be required, depending on the child's strength, endurance, and lifestyle (Neistadt & Crepeau, 1998).

spinal cord injury, paraplegia, tetraplegia

The spinal cord is a cylindrical structure located inside the vertebral column, composed of spinal tracts (white matter) that surround spinal neuronal cell bodies (gray matter). Axons relay sensory and motor information between the gray matter and the spinal nerve roots. The roots are segmentally located and carry information through the foramina of the vertebral column to the dermatomes and myotomes. When the spinal cord is injured, a disruption of the motor, and sensory pathways occurs at the level of the lesion.

Spinal cord injury results in compression caused by contusion or hemorrhage due to laceration or transection of the spinal cord. Contusion causes rapid edematous swelling with increased intradural pressure. Spontaneous improvement happens but with some residual disability (Beers & Berkow, 1999; Yarkony & Chen, 1996). Hemorrhage is usually confined to the cervical central gray matter resulting in signs of lower motor neuron damage, which is usually permanent.

Classification of spinal cord injuries is based on level and type of injury. Four levels are used to describe spinal cord injuries: neurological, motor, sensory, and skeletal. Spinal cord injury is also classified as complete or incomplete based on the presence of sensory or motor function partially preserved below the neurological level. Central cord syndrome, Brown-Sequard syndrome, anterior cord syndrome, and conus medullaris syndrome are specific injuries with unusual impairment of sensory motor function (Hollar, 1995).

Etiology

Spinal cord injuries have many causes. The most common are trauma from motor vehicle accidents (45%), falls (16.8%), sports accidents (16.3%), and violence (Yarkony & Chen, 1996). Diving accidents are also a known cause for spinal cord injury. Normal spinal cord function can also be disturbed by diseases such as tumors, myelomeningocele, syringomyelia, multiple sclerosis, and amyotrophic lateral sclerosis (Adler, 1996). The incidence of SCI ranges from 29.4–50 cases per million (Yarkony & Chen, 1996) and more than 50% are under 30 years of age, the majority being males.

Symptoms

The primary symptoms include:

- Loss of motor function—extent depends on level and type of injury
- Loss of sensation—also depends on level and type of injury
- Pain, including numbness and tingling
- Edema
- Possible respiratory distress
- Changes or loss of function in bladder and bowel functions
- Inability to perform basic or instrumental ADLs
- Spinal shock is a neurovascular shutdown that occurs immediately after a spinal cord injury, characterized by a temporary flaccid paralysis, caused by a suppression of all reflex activity, lasting from hours to months.

Assessment Objectives

The OT will be responsible for assessing occupational performance areas and components. The OT will be involved in assessment and management of the following areas throughout the course of the patient's stay in the acute hospital, rehabilitation setting, and home setting. All areas assessed will be considered in relation to functional performance. Key areas for assessment include various performance areas and skills in order to identify realistic client-centered treatment goals.

Assessment of Performance Areas

- Activities of daily living: BADL and simple IADL skills
- Home management: Home safety, assistive and adaptive devices, environmental modification

161

- Play and leisure skills
- School/educational setting if applicable
- Work/productivity: vocational/prevocational skills

Assessment of Performance Components

Sensory Processing
- Proprioceptive
- Tactile
- Vestibular
- Visual
- Auditory
- Gustatory
- Olfactory

Perceptual Processing
- Stereognosis
- Kinesthesia
- Position in space

Neuromusculoskeletal
- Reflex
- Range of motion
- Muscle tone
- Strength
- Endurance
- Postural control
- Soft tissue integrity

Motor
- Gross coordination
- Bilateral integration
- Motor control
- Praxis
- Fine coordination/dexterity
- Crossing the midline
- Visual-motor integration
- Oral-motor control

Cognitive Integration
- Level of arousal
- Orientation
- Recognition
- Attention span

- Memory
- Initiation of activity
- Problem solving
- Learning
- Generalization

Psychosocial Skills/Psychological Components
- Values
- Interests
- Self-concept
- Role performance
- Interpersonal skills
- Self-control
- Self-expression

Standardized Assessment Tools

- Manual Muscle Test (within limits of precautions)
- Range of Motion test (within limits of precautions)
- Sensory Testing
- Hand function
- Home evaluation for architectural barriers and modification and assistive device/equipment recommendation
- ADL scales
- Occupational performance history
- Work history, job analysis review
- Leisure activities checklist

Standardized Tests
- Functional Independence Measure (FIM℠)
- Klein-Bell ADL Scale
- Barthel Index
- Modified Interest Checklist
- Occupational Performance History Interview
- Jebson Hand function test

Prognosis and Outcome

Prognosis for recovery of neuromuscular function depends mostly on whether the injury is complete or incomplete. In a complete lesion, if there is no sensory or motor function return with the first 48 hours after the injury, motor function is less likely to return. With incomplete lesions, the extent and duration of motor function recovery is difficult to determine. Very often, the longer it takes for recovery to begin, the less likely that it will occur. Modifications may be needed in the physical and social environment to enhance independence. The outcome of rehabilitation also depends on the motivation of the individual notably in making decisions towards the long-term goals and maintaining the focus and intensity of his or her participation throughout the process. Training family members in appropriate assistance of the client may be necessary.

sports injuries See athletic injuries.

stroke See cerebrovascular accident.

tetraplegia See spinal cord injury.

traumatic brain injury

Traumatic brain injury (TBI) can be defined as any injury resulting from a traumatic event that causes direct or indirect damage to the brain. Traumatic injuries to the brain are generally categorized into two different types: a *focal contusion* is a bruising of the brain as a result of a direct blow or impact to the head by an outside force. *Diffuse axonal damage* is damage resulting from a shear force exerted on the axons. A twisting, tearing, or stretching of the axons of the nerve fibers throughout the brain is frequently seen in deceleration accidents.

Etiology

The most common causes in the United States for TBI are high-speed automobile accidents and falls from heights greater than that of the person. Other causes of TBI include: sports injuries, diving injuries, injuries resulting from violence, gunshot wounds, and work-related accidents. Each year more than two million people incur head injuries in the United States (Zasler, Murphy, & Holiday, 1994). Profiles of persons with head injury have been developed with young males (ages 15 to 24) leading high-risk lifestyles demonstrating increased incidence (Winkler, 1995). The next most common profile is that of an elderly person (over 70) with either balance or cognitive deficits, who generally sustains an injury falling in the home environment.

Symptoms

Traumatic brain injury affects all performance areas including ADLs work, and productive activities and play and leisure activities. There is potential for clients to experience deficits in every performance component because of the comprehensive nature of the TBI. Individuals often have motor disturbances with abnormal tone resulting in hemiplegia, paraplegia, triplegia, or quadriplegia. Impairments in range of motion (ROM), postural control, and poor motor control may be present. Sensory disturbances may be determined. Cognitive deficits in level of arousal, orientation, attention, memory, sequencing, and organizing may also be noted in TBI. Clients may be unable to problem-solve or to learn new information effectively. Other symptoms may include: deficits in visual perception, spatial relations, position in space, depth perception, and figure ground. Clients will frequently have impairment in their ability to manage language, interfering with their ability to display self-expression and socialization skills. Clients can easily become overwhelmed and frequently demonstrate difficulty with behavior and emotion management and coping skills (Winkler, 1995).

Assessment Objectives

The OT will assess occupational performance areas and components. The areas an OT evaluates are frequently determined by the level of recovery a patient has reached and by the type of setting in which the clinician practices. All areas assessed will be considered in relation to functional performance. Key areas for assessment include various performance areas and skills in order to identify realistic client-centered treatment goals.

Assessment of Performance Areas

- Activities of daily living: BADL and IADL skills
- Home management: Home safety, assistive devices, and environmental modification
- Work and productivity: Educational, prevocational, and vocational
- Play and leisure

Assessment of Performance Components

Sensory Processing
- Proprioceptive
- Tactile

- Vestibular
- Visual
- Auditory
- Gustatory
- Olfactory

Perceptual Processing
- Stereognosis
- Kinesthesia
- Position in space
- Right-left discrimination
- Form constancy
- Visual closure
- Figure ground
- Body scheme
- Depth perception
- Spatial relations
- Topographical orientation

Neuromusculoskeletal
- Range of motion
- Reflex
- Muscle tone
- Strength
- Endurance
- Postural control
- Postural alignment
- Soft tissue integrity

Motor
- Gross coordination
- Bilateral integration
- Motor control
- Praxis
- Fine coordination/dexterity
- Laterality
- Crossing the midline
- Visual-motor integration
- Oral-motor control

Cognitive Integration
- Level of arousal
- Orientation

- Recognition
- Attention span
- Memory
- Sequencing
- Categorization
- Initiation of activity
- Termination of activity
- Concept formation
- Spatial operations
- Problem solving
- Learning
- Generalization

Psychosocial Skills/Psychological Components

- Values
- Interests
- Self-concept
- Social conduct
- Role performance
- Interpersonal skills
- Self-control
- Self-expression
- Time management

Standardized Assessment Tools

- Coma/Near Coma Scale (CNCS)
- Coma Recovery Scale (CRS)
- Sensory Stimulation Assessment Measure (SSAM)
- Western Sensory Stimulation Profile (WNSSP)
- Awareness Questionnaire
- Self-Awareness Deficits Interview
- Community Integration Questionnaire (CIQ)
- Functional Independence Measure (FIM^{SM})
- Assessment of Motor and Process Skills (AMPS)
- The Cognitive Assessment of Minnesota (CAM)
- Lowenstein Occupational Therapy Cognitive Assessment (LOTCA)
- Head Injury Symptom Checklist
- Goniometer
- Dynamometer
- Pinch meter

Prognosis and Outcome

Prognosis for persons who sustain TBI is dependent upon several things. Client age, the size and location of the injury, the type of injury, the level of consciousness at the time of the injury, and the length of coma if loss of consciousness occurs are all contributing factors to the clinician's determination of prognosis in TBI. The Glasgow Scale is a scale generally used at the scene of the accident and frequently during emergent care and acute care phases to monitor a client's level of consciousness. Prognostic indicators that support a positive outcome include (Katz, 1992):

• Young age
• A small lesion in a noncritical part of the brain
• Focal rather than diffuse injury
• Loss of consciousness post-injury for more than 1 day

vision See low vision.

weakness See deconditioned/generalized debility or weakness.

Appendix A
Acronyms

ACIS	Assessment of Communication and Interactional Skills
ACLS	Allen Cognitive Level Scale
AD	Alzheimer's disease
ADC	adult day care
ADHD	attention deficit/hyperactive disorder
ADL	activities of daily living
ALS	amyotrophic lateral sclerosis
AMC	arthrogryposis multiplex congenita
AMPS	Assessment of Motor and Process Skills
APA	American Psychiatric Association
BADL	basic activity of daily living
BOTMP	Bruininks-Oseretsky Test of Motor Proficiency
BSID-II	Bayley Scales of Infant Development-II
CAM	The Cognitive Assessment of Minnesota
CASE	Cognitive Adaptive Skills Evaluation
CFS	chronic fatigue syndrome
CIQ	Community Integration Questionnaire
CJD	Creutzfeldt-Jakob disease
CNC	Coma/Near Coma Scale
CNS	central nervous system
COMPS	Clinical Observations of Motor and Postural Skills
COPD	chronic obstructive pulmonary disease
COPM	Canadian Occupational Performance Measure
COTNAB	The Chessington Occupational Therapy Neurological Assessment Battery
CP	cerebral palsy
CRS	Coma Recovery Scale
CVA	cerebrovascular accident
DBTSI	DeGangi-Berk Test of Sensory Integration
DD	developmental disability
DNA	deoxyribonucleic acid
DSM-IV	*Diagnostic and Statistical Manual-IV*
EMS	emergency medical services

FAE	fetal alcohol effect
FAS	fetal alcohol syndrome
FIM	Functional Independence Measure
FTII	Fagan Test of Infant Intelligence
GCS	Glasgow Coma Scale
GDS	Geriatric Depression Scale
ICP	intracranial pressure
ICS	Innsbruck Coma Scale
ICU	intensive care unit
IEP	Individual Education Plan
IQ	intelligence quotient
KELS	Kohlman Evaluation of Living Skills
LBP	low back pain
LD	learning disability
LMN	lower motor neuron
LOTCA	Lowenstein Occupational Therapy Cognitive Assessment
MAI	Motor Assessment of Infants
MAP	Miller Assessment for Preschoolers
MD	muscular dystrophy
MEAMS	Middlesex Elderly Assessment of Mental Status
MEDLS	Milwaukee Evaluation of Daily Living Skills
MG	myasthenia gravis
MID	multi-infarct dementia
MMDT	Minnesota Manual Dexterity Test
MMSE	Mini-Mental State Exam
MMT	manual muscle test
MPQ	McGill Pain Questionnaire
MR	mental retardation
MRMT	Minnesota Rate of Manipulation Test
MS	multiple sclerosis
MSRT	Minnesota Spatial Relations Test
MVPT-R	Motor-Free Visual Perception Test—Revised
MVPT-V	Motor-Free Visual Perception Test—Vertical
NIA	National Institute on Aging
NIDA	National Institute on Drug Abuse

NRS	Numerical Rating Scale
OA	osteoarthritis
OCAIRS	Occupational Case Analysis and Interview Rating Scale
OPHI-II	Occupational Performance History Interview II
ORIF	open reduction internal fixation
OT	occupational therapist
PAT	Pain Apperception Test
PDMS	Peabody Developmental Motor Scales
PTA	post-traumatic amnesia
PVD	peripheral vascular disease
RA	rheumatoid arthritis
ROM	range of motion
SCI	spinal cord injury
SDAT	senile dementia of the Alzheimer's type
SI	sensory integration
SOTOF	Structural Observational Test of Function
SSAM	Sensory Stimulation Assessment Measure
SSSQ	Street Survival Skills Questionnaire
TBI	traumatic brain injury
TBSA	total body surface area
THR or THA	total hip replacement or total hip arthroplasty
TIME	Toddler and Infant Motor Evaluation
TSCS	Tennessee Self-Concept Scale
TSFI	Test of Sensory Function in Infants
TVMS-R	Test of Visual Motor Skills-Revised
UMN	upper motor neuron
UT-III	Uniform Terminology III
VAS	Visual Analog Scale
VOT	Hooper Visual Organization Test
VRS	Verbal Rating Scale
WNSSP	Western Sensory Stimulation Profile

Appendix B
Home Evaluation

Planning for the client's discharge should begin on day one of the therapy process. To ensure return to the highest functional performance level and to ensure client safety, a home visit for the purpose of assessing the physical living environment and the client's functioning within that setting is generally favorable. Frequently, home assessments are carried out to determinine the efficacy of current living environments, particularly for older adults when dementia is a consideration.

A home assessment should be carried out to facilitate the client's maximum safety and independence in the living environment. Ideally, the client and his or her family members are present during the visit. Either the occupational or physical therapist is well-suited to perform the home assessment. It is essential to interview the client to determine the significant roles and goals of the individual, as well as to determine the client's and the family's expectations. An assessment of the client's willingness and financial ability to make modifications in the home should also be determined.

A comprehensive home assessment can be multifocal and include various screening tools such as ROM screen, vision screen, nutrition screen, Geriatric Depression Scale (GDS), Mini-Mental State Exam (MMSE), Get Up and Go Test for Balance, Functional Activities of Daily Living Screen, home hazard and safety screen, medication management and administration screen, review of past medical history, a review of family history, and survey of current financial and social status (including involvement with any social service agencies such as Senior Services, Meals-on-Wheels, community day care, or respite care services).

During the performance evaluation, the therapist should constantly be observing safety factors, ease of mobility and performance, and limitations presented by the environment. At the conclusion of the evaluation, the therapist can develop a list of problems, modifications recommended, and a description of safety equipment and assistive devices. Also at the end of the assessment, the therapist writes a report including information describing the client's performance and summarizing the information on the evaluation form. It is essential to include a concise summary of the environmental barriers and the client's functional and safety limitations. Recomnendations should be written using specific terms and clear descriptions of size, type, building specifications, costs (round figures), and available resources in the community.

Many therapists use adapted versions of various assessments and screening tools as a successful means of collecting relevant data during home evaluation visits. Most of these tools are not standardized but do provide a basis of information valuable for team decision-making.

- Nutrition screen
- Geriatric Depression Scale
- Mini-Mental State Examination
- Tinetti Screen for Gait and Balance
- Clock Drawing Test
- Screen of medication management and administration
- Home hazard and safety screen

f time permits during the home assessment, the therapist may find t helpful to administer the Assessment of Motor and Process Skills (AMPS). This may add another 45–60 minutes to the visit and should be scheduled accordingly.

The therapist should include recommendations about the client remaining in his or her existing home or returning home after discharge. In most cases, the team will appreciate the insight of the therapist. The unique perspective of one who has actually seen the client's home adds rich information to the decision-making process. If there is a question about the client's ability to remain in his or her current residence independently, the home assessment summary should include a clear indication of the functional skills that the client will need to return home as well as those skills currently lacking.

Appendix C

Occupational Therapy Assessments: Tests and Resources

This appendix presents information on a wide range of assessment tests in occupational therapy. The function of each test is briefly discussed, followed by information on how to learn more or to obtain the assessment. This appendix is adapted and updated from *Occupational Therapy Assessment Tools: An Annotated Index* (2nd ed.) by I. E. Asher. Bethesda, MD: American Occupational Therapy Association (1996).

Allen Cognitive Level Test (ACL)

Function:

- Clinical instrument for assessment of cognitive disability
- Use of simple tools and manual dexterity tasks to examine cognitive function according to the author's theoretical hierarchy of cognitive functioning levels

Source: S&S Worldwide, P.O. Box 513, Colchester, CT 06415-0513 Telephone: 800-243-9232; Fax: 800-566-6678.

Assessment of Communication and Interaction Skills (ACIS)

Function:

- Measurement of an individual's personal communication and group interaction skills
- Assessment takes place during involvement in routine daily activities performance

Source: Model of Human Occupation Clearinghouse, University of Illinois at Chicago, Department of Occupational Therapy (M/C 811), College of Applied Health Sciences, 1919 West Taylor Street, Chicago, IL 60612-7249. Telephone: 312-996-6901; Fax 312-413-0256.

Assessment of Motor and Process Skills (AMPS)

Function:

- An objective assessment of motor and process skills in the context of performing familiar functional tasks
- Tasks assessed are chosen by the individual
- Identifies the causes of IADL limitations
- Assists with treatment planning
- May predict performance ability in other areas of IADL

Source: Anne G. Fisher, ScD, OTR/L, FAOTA, AMPS Project, Occupational Therapy Building, Colorado State University, Fort Collins, CO 80523. Telephone: 970-491-6299.

Barthel Index

Function:

- Simple index of independence used to assess change in functional status

Source: Mahoney, F. I., & Barthel, D. W. (1965). Functional evaluation: The Barthel Index. *Maryland State Medical Journal, 14,* 61–65.

Bayley Infant Neurodevelopmental Screener (BINS)

Function:

- Used as a screening tool to identify infants with neurological impairments or developmental delay

Source: The Psychological Corporation, 19500 Bulverde Road, San Antonio, TX 78259-3701. Telephone: 800-872-1726. Fax: 800-232-1223.

Bayley Scales of Infant Development, 2nd Edition (BSID-II)

Function:

- Designed to evaluate mental, motor, and social development in early childhood
- May be used to diagnose developmental delay and to plan intervention

Source: The Psychological Corporation, 19500 Bulverde Road, San Antonio, TX 78259-3701. Telephone: 800-872-1726. Fax: 800-232-1223.

Blessed Dementia Rating Scale

Function:

- Basic activities of daily living are assessed
- Attempts to quantify the degree of cognitive and personality change demonstrated in people with dementia

Source: Blessed, G., Thomlinson, B. E., & Roth, M. (1968). The association between quantitative measures of dementia and of senile change in the cerebral gray matter of elderly subjects. *British Journal of Psychiatry, 114,* 797–811.

Bruininks-Oseretsky Test of Motor Proficiency

Function:

- Measures gross and fine motor skills

- Provides a comprehensive index of motor proficiency
- This instrument can be successfully used by clinicians, educators, and in the research domain

Source: American Guidance Service, Inc., 4201 Woodland Road, Circle Pines, MN 55014. Telephone: 800-328-2560; Fax: 612-786-9077.

Canadian Occupational Performance Measure, 2nd Edition (COPM)

Function:

- A client-centered outcome measure
- Utilizes client perceptions of occupational performance and satisfaction with performance levels to identify problem areas
- May be used to assist in development of treatment interventions

Source: Canadian Association of Occupational Therapists, CTTC Building, Suite 3400, 1125 Colonel By Drive, Ottawa, ON K1S 5R1 Canada. Telephone: 800-434-2268.

The Chessington OT Neurological Assessment Battery (COTNAB)

Function:

- Designed to assess neurological clients specifically in areas of functional ability
- Visual perception, constructional ability, sensorimotor ability, and the ability to follow instructions are included as parts of the assessment

Source: Nottingham Rehab Limited, Nottingham, England. Distributed in the U.S.A. by North Coast Medical, 18305 Sutter Boulevard, Morgan Hill, CA 95037-2842. Telephone: 800-821-9319; Fax: 877-213-9300.

Clinical Observations of Motor and Postural Skills (COMPS)

Function:

- Clinical observation techniques are used in this screening tool to identify motor problems having a postural component in the pediatric population

Source: Therapy Skill Builders, a division of the Psychological Corporation, 19500 Bulverde Road, San Antonio, TX 78259-3701. Telephone: 800-872-1726. Fax: 800-232-1223.

Cognitive Assessment of Minnesota

Function:

- Screens a wide range of cognitive skills
- Identification of general problem areas and development of treatment intervention
- Used as a baseline instrument or as a tool for measuring cognitive change over time

Source: Therapy Skill Builders, a division of the Psychological Corporation, 19500 Bulverde Road, San Antonio, TX 78259-3701. Telephone: 800-872-1726. Fax: 800-232-1223.

Coping Inventory

Function:

- Measures adaptive and maladaptive coping habits, skills, and behaviors used by children
- Coping skills needed for school, daily activities, and in the community are assessed

Source: Scholastic Testing Service, Inc., 480 Meyer Road, Bensenville, IL 60106-1617. Telephone: 800-642-6787; Fax: 708-766-8054.

Crawford Small Parts Dexterity Test

Function:

- Measures fine hand coordination for vocational testing
- Primarily designed to predict job performance in industry
- Test has also been used to assess manual dexterity

Source: The Psychological Corporation, 19500 Bulverde Road, San Antonio, TX 78259-3701. Telephone: 800-872-1726. Fax: 800-232-1223.

DeGangi-Berk Test of Sensory Integration (DBTSI)

Function:

- Measure of sensory integration in preschoolers
- Designed to detect sensory integrative dysfunction
- Used as a screening tool and for development of diagnoses

Source: Western Psychological Services, 12031 Wilshire Boulevard, Los Angeles, CA 90025. Telephone: 800-648-8857; Fax: 310-478-7838.

Denver II

Function:

- By giving an overview of the child's development, this tool is designed to provide early identification of children at risk of developmental deficits

Source: Denver Developmental Materials, Inc. (1967, 1975, 1989), P.O. Box 371075, Denver, CO 80237. Telephone: 800-419-4729.

Developmental Test of Visual Perception, 2nd Edition (DTVP-2)

Function:

- Deficits in visual perception and visual-motor integration are screened and identified
- Degree of impairment and the need for intervention can be determined using this tool

Source: PRO-ED, Inc., 8700 Shoal Creek Boulevard, Austin, TX 78757. Telephone: 800-897-3202; Fax: 800-397-7633.

Developmental Test of Visual-Motor Integration—3rd Revision (VMI) (1967, revised 1982, 1989)

Function:

- A classroom-screening tool for early identification of learning deficits

Source: Modern Curriculum Press, 135 S. Mt. Zion Road, Lebanon, IN 46052. Telephone: 800-526-9907.

Dysphagia Evaluation Protocol (1996)

Function:

- Designed as a clinical assessment tool to provide an objective measure of swallow function
- Used as a screening tool to identify clients who may benefit from further assessment of the swallow mechanism, including oral and pharyngeal components

Source: Therapy Skill Builders, a division of the Psychological Corporation, 19500 Bulverde Road, San Antonio, TX 78259-3701. Telephone: 800-872-1726. Fax: 800-232-1223.

Early Coping Inventory

Function:

- Measures coping, and coping-related behaviors demonstrated by infants and toddlers in the context of everyday life
- Educational and therapeutic intervention strategies can be developed as an outcome

Source: Scholastic Testing Service, Inc., 480 Meyer Road, Bensenville, IL 60610-8054. Telephone: 800-642-6787; Fax: 708-766-8054.

Functional Assessment Staging (FAST)

Function:

- Tool developed to assess the clinically identifiable stages of dementia

Source: Reisberg, B., Sclan, S. G., Franssen, E., Kluger, A., & Ferris, S. (1994). Dementia staging in chronic care populations. *Alzheimer Disease and Associated Disorders*, 8(Suppl. 1), S188–S205.

Functional Independence Measure (FIM^SM) and Functional Independence Measure for Children (Wee FIM^SM)

Function:

- Designed to provide a clinical evaluation of the client
- Group data designed to determine rehabilitation outcomes may be achieved
- Measures functional status and the impact of disability on the individual

Sources: Uniform Data System for Medical Rehabilitation, 270 Northpointe Parkway, Suite 300, Amherst, NY 14228. Telephone: 716-817-7800; Fax: 716-568-0037; e-mail: info@udsmr.org.

Global Deterioration Scale (GDS)

Function:

- Measures the stages of primary degenerative dementia and age-associated memory impairment
- Designed to allow follow-up on the onset and progression of the disease process
- Allows for the measurement of levels of cognitive and functional deterioration

Source: Reisberg, B., Ferris, S. H., DeLeon, M. J., & Crook, T. (1982). The Global Deterioration Scale for assessment of primary degenerative dementia. *American Journal of Psychiatry*, *139*, 1136–1139.

Hooper Visual Organization Test (VOT)

Function:

- Readily administered in clinical and research settings
- Measures the ability to integrate visual stimuli
- Considered for use in a comprehensive neurological battery

Source: Western Psychological Services, 12031 Wilshire Blvd., Los Angeles, CA 90025. Telephone: 800-648-8857; Fax: 310-478-7838.

Interest Checklist

Function:

- Measures the interest patterns and involvement of an individual during his or her lifetime

Source: Modified Interest Checklist available from Model of Human Occupation Clearinghouse, University of Illinois at Chicago, Department of Occupational Therapy (M/C 811), College of Applied Health Sciences, 1919 West Taylor Street, Chicago, IL 60612-7249. Telephone: 312-996-6901; Fax: 312-413-0256.

Jebson Hand Function Test

Function:

- A simple and effective test of hand dexterity
- Functional and manual activities are included as part of the test
- May be used to determine treatment intervention strategies and to measure effectiveness of treatment intervention

Sources: The test kit may be purchased from Sammons/Preston Inc., P.O. Box 50710, Bolingbrook, IL 60440-5071. Telephone: 800-323-5547; Fax: 800-547-4333.

Jebson, R. H., Taylor, N., Trieschmann, R. B., Trotter, M. J., & Howard, L. A. (1969, June). An objective and standardized test of hand function. *Archives of Physical Medicine and Rehabilitation*, 311–319.

Kitchen Task Assessment (KTA)

Function:

- Measures organizational, planning, and judgment skills
- Common kitchen tasks are utilized

Source: Baum, C., & Edwards, D. (1993). Cognitive performance in senile dementia of the Alzheimer's type: The Kitchen Task Assessment. *American Journal of Occupational Therapy, 47,* 431–436.

Klein-Bell Activities of Daily Living Scale

Function:

- An assessment of the client's current functional level in ADL skills
- Functional progress can be measured, documented, and communicated to the care team
- Can be used to develop treatment interventions and strategies

Source: Health Sciences Center for Educational Resources, University of Washington, T-281 Health Sciences Building, Box 357161, Seattle, WA 98195-7161. Telephone: 206-685-1158; Fax: 206-543-8051.

Kohlman Evaluation of Living Skills (KELS), 3rd edition

Function:

- Readily administered, requires minimal set-up
- Designed to assess basic skills for living outside of an institution
- Can assist in identifying levels of functional independence
- Can be utilized to assist a care team in determining appropriate living environments for a client

Source: American Occupational Therapy Association, Inc., 4720 Montgomery Lane, P.O. Box 31220, Bethesda, MD 20824-1220. Telephone: 301-652-2682; Fax: 301-652-7711.

Lowenstein Occupational Therapy Cognitive Assessment (LOTCA)

Function:

- Developed for use with neurologically involved clients
- A battery of concise assessments that are client-centered
- Cognitive function is assessed

Source: Developed by Lowenstein Rehabilitation Hospital, Israel. Published by Maddak, Inc., 661 Route 23 South, Wayne, NJ 07470. Telephone: 973-628-7600; Fax: 973-305-0841.

The Middlesex Elderly Assessment of Mental State (MEAMS)

Function:

- To detect impairment in major cognitive skills areas in the elderly
- May be used to distinguish between functional impairment and organically derived impairments

Source: Published by Thames Valley Test Company, Suffolk, England. Distributed by National Rehabilitation Services, 117 North Elm Street, P.O. Box 1247, Gaylord, MI 49735. Telephone: 989-732-3866; Fax: 989-732-6164.

Miller Assessment for Preschoolers (MAP)

Function:

- Used to determine developmental status and identify moderate developmental delays
- Found to be statistically sound
- A comprehensive and concise tool

Sources: The Psychological Corporation, 19500 Bulverde Road, San Antonio, TX 78259-3701. Telephone: 800-872-1726. Fax: 800-232-1223.

Miller, L. (1983). MAP: A review. *American Journal of Occupational Therapy, 37*(5), 333–340.

Milwaukee Evaluation of Daily Living Skills (MEDLS)

Function:

- Developed to provide a standard, quantifiable measurement of daily living skills
- Primarily utilized with the lower-functioning, long-term psychiatric client
- Easy to administer and score, providing an effective means for treatment planning and goal development

Source: Leonardelli, C. A. (1988). *The Milwaukee Evaluation of Daily Living Skills: Evaluation in long-term psychiatric care.* Thorofare, NJ: Slack.

Mini-Mental State Exam (MMSE)

Function:

- Short, simple-to-administer quantifiable measure of cognitive function
- Used clinically and routinely for examination and tracking of mental status

Source: Folstein, M. F., Folstein, S. E., & McHugh, P. R. (1975). Mini mental state: A practical method for grading the cognitive state of patients for the clinician. *Journal of Psychiatric Research, 12,* 189–198.

Minnesota Manual Dexterity Test (MMDT)

Function:

- Manual dexterity and gross eye-hand coordination are measured quantitatively
- Developed for use in evaluation of vocational potential
- Performance in general semi-skilled tasks is assessed

Source: Lafayette Instrument Co., 3700 Sagamore Parkway North, P.O. Box 5729, Lafayette, IN 47904. Telephone: 800-428-7545; Fax: 765-423-4111.

Minnesota Rate of Manipulation Tests (MRMT)

Function:

- Manual dexterity and speed of upper extremity movements are measured during rapid eye-hand coordination tasks

Source: American Guidance Service, Inc., 4201 Woodland Road, Circle Pines, MN 55014. Telephone: 800-328-2560; Fax: 612-786-9077

Minnesota Spatial Relations Test (MSRT)

Function:

- Spatial visualization ability is determined by measuring speed and accuracy of eye-hand coordination movements during activities involving placement of three-dimensional objects

Source: American Guidance Service, Inc., 4201 Woodland Road, Circle Pines, MN 55014. Telephone: 800-328-2560; Fax: 612-786-9077.

Motor-Free Visual Perception Test—Revised (MVPT-R)

Function:

- Developed to provide a quick and simple assessment of visual perception with motor involvement of the subject eliminated
- Used as a screening tool and for diagnostic purposes

Source: Academic Therapy Publications, 20 Commercial Blvd., Novato, CA 94949-6120. Telephone: 800-422-7249; Fax: 888-287-9975.

Motor-Free Visual Perception Test-Vertical (MVPT-V)

Function:

- Developed to provide a quick and simple assessment of visual perception with motor involvement of the subject eliminated
- Used as a screening tool and for diagnostic purposes

Source: Academic Therapy Publications, 20 Commercial Blvd., Novato, CA 94949-6120. Telephone: 800-422-7249; Fax: 888-287-9975.

Occupational Case Analysis Interview and Rating Scale

Function:

- Designed for assistance in discharge planning and to aid the client in community reentry and adjustment
- Evaluates the client's abilities in occupational adaptation

Source: Slack Incorporated, 6900 Grove Road, Thorofare, NJ 08086. Telephone: 800-257-8290; Fax: 800-853-5991.

Occupational Performance History Interview (OPHI)

Function:

- Developed to gather a history of the client's work, play, and self-care performance
- Based on the Model of Human Occupation
- May offer information of how the client perceives life

Sources: American Occupational Therapy Association, Inc., 4720 Montgomery Lane, P.O. Box 31220, Bethesda, MD 20824-1220. Telephone: 301-652-2682; Fax: 301-652-7711.

Kielhofner, G. (1995). *A model of human occupation: Theory and application* (2nd ed.). Baltimore: Williams & Wilkins.

Kielhofner, G., Henry, A., Whalens, D., & Rogers, E. S. (1991). A generalizability study of the Occupational Performance History Interview. *Occupational Therapy Journal of Research, 11,* 292–306.

Pain Apperception Test (PAT)

Function:

- Developed to measure the psychological variables involved in the pain experience
- May be of assistance in determining differences in pain perception among various cohorts

Source: Western Psychological Services, 12031 Wilshire Boulevard, Los Angeles, CA 90025. Telephone: 800-648-8857; Fax: 310-478-7838.

Peabody Developmental Motor Scales (PDMS)

Function:

- Assessment scales accommodate the needs of a severely disabled population
- Developed as an evaluation of gross and fine motor development in children
- Assists in determining levels of skill development and to identify skill deficiencies
- Valuable for planning intervention and remediation strategies

Source: Riverside Publishing Co., 425 Spring Lake Drive, Itasca, IL 60143-2079. Telephone: 800-323-9540; Fax: 630-467-7192.

Play Observation

Function:

- Utilizing standardized conditions, data on children's behaviors during play and at other times can be measured
- Behaviors are described in relation to the subject's physical and social environment during the assessment

Source: Kalverboer, A. (1977). A measurement of play: Clinical applications. In B. Tizard & D. Harvey (Eds.), *Biology of play*. Philadelphia: Lippincott.

Purdue Pegboard

Function:

- Primarily intended as a vocational assessment for industrial jobs, this assessment has a variety of clinical applications
- Developed as a simple, readily administered measurement of hand dexterity during fingertip tasks

- Assessment of the entire upper extremity can be achieved as well

Sources: Available from Lafayette Instrument Company, 3700 Sagamore Parkway North, P.O. Box 5729, Lafayette, IN 47904. Telephone: 800-428-7545; Fax: 765-423-4111.

Mathiowetz, V., Rogers, S. L., Dowe-Keval, M., Donahoe, L., & Rennells, C. (1986). The Purdue Pegboard: Norms for 14- to 19-year-olds. *American Journal of Occupational Therapy, 40*(3), 174–179.

Sensory Integration Inventory—Revised, for Individuals with Disabilities

Function:

- Developed as screening tool for individuals with developmental disabilities who may be presenting with impairments in sensory integrative (SI) function
- Assists in identifying clients for whom SI treatment may be beneficial
- Acts as a screener of those clients who likely do not have SI dysfunction

Source: PDP Products, 14524 61st Street Ct. N., Stillwater, MN 55082. Telephone: 651-439-8865; Fax: 651-439-0421.

Sensory Integration and Praxis Tests (SIPT) (1989)

Function:

- The tests are utilized to assess praxis, sensory processing, and the integration of sensory and perceptual systems
- A diagnostic and screening tool developed to assist the clinician in distinguishing between normal children and children presenting with sensory integrative and learning deficits
- Valuable for treatment planning and development of intervention strategies

Sources: Available from Western Psychological Services, 12031 Wilshire Boulevard, Los Angeles, CA 90025. Telephone: 800-648-8857; Fax: 310-478-7838.

Training and certification through Sensory Integration International, P.O. Box 5339, Torrance, CA 90510-5339. Telephone: 310-787-8805; Fax: 310-787-8130.

Street Survival Skills Questionnaire (SSSQ)

Function:

- Used as a tool for predicting successful community placement and for vocational placement

- Measures levels of specific community-related adaptive skills

Source: McCarron-Dial Systems, P.O. Box 45628, Dallas, TX 75245. Telephone: 214-634-2863.

Structured Observational Test of Function (SOTOF)

Function:

- Developed as a screening tool for clients with neuropsychological impairments
- Designed to provide detailed information on functional status, as determined by structured assessment of activities of daily living
- Baseline information can be used for treatment planning

Source: NFER-Nelson Publishing Company Ltd., Unit 28, Bramble Road, Swindon, Wiltshire, SN2 8EZ, England. Telephone: +44 (0) 20 8996 8445; Fax: +44 (0)20 8996 3660. E-mail: international@nfer-nelson.co.uk

Tennessee Self-Concept Scale—Revised (TSCSR)

Function:

- Provides an assessment of self-concept in a readily administered format
- Used in clinical assessment, research, personnel selection and evaluation, and for diagnostic purposes

Source: Western Psychological Services, 12031 Wilshire Boulevard, Los Angeles, CA 90025. Telephone: 800-648-8857; Fax: 310-478-7838.

Test of Sensory Functions in Infants (TSFI)

Function:

- Provides screening of sensory integrative dysfunction in infants
- Recommended for use in conjunction with a battery of other evaluations, this tool assists the user in determining infants at risk for learning disorders

Source: Western Psychological Services, 12031 Wilshire Boulevard, Los Angeles, CA 90025. Telephone: 800-648-8857; Fax: 310-478-7838.

Test of Visual-Motor Skills (TVMS) and Test of Visual-Motor Skills: Upper Level Adolescents and Adults (TVMS: UL)

Function:

- Measures the child or adult's ability to visually perceive nonlanguage forms and transfer what is perceived through hand function tasks

- A valuable tool for developing treatment planning strategies

Source: Psychological and Educational Publications, Inc., 1477 Rollins Road, Burlingame, CA 94010. Telephone: 800-523-5775; Fax: 800-447-0907.

The T.I.M.E. Toddler and Infant Motor Evaluation

Function:

- Measures motor abilities and quality of movement in children
- Determines motor delays or deficiencies
- Valuable in determining appropriate treatment interventions

Source: Therapy Skill Builders, a division of the Psychological Corporation, 19500 Bulverde Road, San Antonio, TX 78259-3701. Telephone: 800-872-1726. Fax: 800-232-1223.

Vineland Adaptive Behavior Scales, Revised (VABS)

Function:

- Measures an individual's ability to perform daily life activities and to get along with others

Source: American Guidance Service, Inc., 4201 Woodland Road, Circle Pines, MN 55014. Telephone: 800-328-2560; Fax: 612-786-9077.

Worker Role Interview (WRI)

Function:

- May be utilized as a component of the initial rehabilitation therapy assessment
- Developed to determine specific variables that may influence an individual's ability to return to the workplace

Sources: Distributed by Model of Human Occupation Clearinghouse, University of Illinois at Chicago, Department of Occupational Therapy (M/C 811), College of Applied Health Sciences, 1919 West Taylor Street, Chicago, IL 60612-7249. Telephone: 312-996-6901; Fax: 312-413-0256.

Biernacki, S. (1993). Reliability of the Worker Role Interview. *American Journal of Occupational Therapy, 47,* 797–803.

Kielhofner, G. (1995). *A model of human occupation: Theory and application* (2nd ed.). Baltimore: Williams & Wilkins.

Appendix D
Table of Muscles

Muscles	Origin	Insertion	Innervation	Action
Muscles of the Back				
Superficial Muscles				
Trapezius	External occipital protuberance, superior nucal line, ligamentum nuchae, spines of C7–T12	Spine of scapula, acromion, and lateral third of clavicle	Spinal accessory n., C3–C4	Adducts, rotates, elevates, and depresses scapula
Levator scapulae	Transverse processes of C1–C4	Medial border of scapula	Nerves to levator scapulae, C3–C4; dorsal scapular n.	Elevates scapula
Rhomboid minor	Spines of C7–T1	Root of spine of scapula	Dorsal scapular n., C5	Adducts scapula
Rhomboid major	Spines of T2–T5	Medial border of scapula	Dorsal scapular n.	Adducts scapula
Latissimus dorsi	Spines of T5–T12, thoracodorsal fascia, iliac crest, ribs 9–12	Floor of bicipital groove of humerus	Thoracodorsal n.	Adducts, extends, and rotates arm medially

Muscles	Origin	Insertion	Innervation	Action
Intermediate Muscles				
Serratus posterior–superior	Ligamentum nuchae, supraspinal ligament, and spines of C7–T3	Upper border of ribs 2–5	Intercostal n., T1–T4	Elevates ribs
Serratus posterior–inferior	Supraspinous ligament and spines of T11–L3	Lower border of ribs 9–12	Intercostal n., T9–T12	Depresses ribs
Deep Muscles (Intrinsics)				
Superficial Layer of Deep Muscles (Spinotransverse Group)				
Splenius capitis	Inferior half of ligamentum nuchae, spinous processes of T1–T6	Lateral aspect of mastoid process, lateral third of superior nuchal line	Dorsal rami of inferior cervical n.	Alone, it laterally flexes and rotates head and neck to same side; it works with the other splenius muscle to extend the head and neck
Splenius cervicis	Inferior half of ligamentum nuchae, spinous processes of T1–T6	Posterior tubercles of transverse processes of C1–C4	Dorsal rami of inferior cervical n.	Alone, it laterally flexes and rotates head and neck to same side; it works with the other splenius muscle to extend the head and neck

(continued)

189

(continued)

Intermediate Layer of Deep Muscles (Sacrospinalis or Erector Spinae Group)

Muscles	Origin	Insertion	Innervation	Action
Iliocostalis (Lateral column)	Posterior part of iliac crest, posterior aspect of sacrum, sacroiliac ligaments, and sacral and inferior lumbar spinous processes	Angles of the ribs, cervical transverse processes	Dorsal rami of spinal n.	Bilaterally, they extend the head and vertebral column; unilaterally, they laterally flex the head or vertebral column
Longissimus (Intermediate column)	Posterior part of iliac crest, posterior aspect of sacrum, sacroiliac ligaments, and sacral and inferior lumbar spinous processes	Transverse processes of thoracic and cervical vertebrae, mastoid process	Dorsal rami of spinal n.	Same as above; also, the longissimus capitis rotates the head to the same side
Spinalis (Medial column)	Posterior part of iliac crest, posterior aspect of sacrum, sacroiliac ligaments, and sacral and inferior lumbar spinous processes	Spinous processes from lumbar to thoracic region	Dorsal rami of spinal n.	Bilaterally, they extend the head and vertebral column; unilaterally, they laterally flex the head or vertebral column

Muscles	Origin	Insertion	Innervation	Action
Deep Layer of Deep Muscles (Transversospinalis Group)				
Semispinalis thoracis	Transverse processes	Thoracic and cervical spinous processes	Dorsal rami of cervical spinal n.	Bilaterally, extends the cervical and thoracic regions of vertebral column; unilaterally, rotates toward the opposite side
Semispinalis cervicis	Transverse processes	Thoracic and cervical spinous processes	Dorsal rami of cervical spinal n.	Bilaterally, extends the cervical and thoracic regions of vertebral column; unilaterally, rotates toward the opposite side
Semispinalis capitis	Transverse processes of T1–T6	Medial half of area between superior and inferior nuchal line on occipital bone	Dorsal rami of cervical spinal n.	Bilaterally, extends the head; unilaterally, rotates toward the opposite side

(continued)

(continued)

Muscles	Origin	Insertion	Innervation	Action
Multifidus	Laminae of S4-C2	Span 1–3 vertebrae before inserting in spinous processes	Dorsal rami of cervical spinal n.	Bilaterally, extend the trunk and stabilize the vertebral column; unilaterally, flex the trunk laterally and rotate it to the opposite side
Rotators	Transverse processes	Base of the spinous process superior to vertebra of origin	Dorsal rami of cervical spinal n.	Rotate the superior vertebra to the opposite side and stabilize it
Segmental Muscles				
Interspinales	Spinous processes	Adjacent spinous processes	Dorsal rami of cervical spinal n.	Extend the vertebral column
Intertransversarii	Transverse processes	Adjacent transverse processes	Ventral and dorsal rami of cervical spinal n.	Bilaterally, extend the vertebral column; unilaterally, laterally flex the superior vertebra
Levator costarum	Transverse processes	Rib just inferior to vertebra of origin	Dorsal rami of spinal n.	Elevate the ribs during inspiration

Muscles	Origin	Insertion	Innervation	Action
Suboccipital Muscles				
Rectus capitis posterior major	Spine of axis	Lateral portion of inferior nuchal line	Suboccipital n.	Extends, rotates, and flexes head laterally
Rectus capitis posterior minor	Posterior tubercle of atlas	Occipital bone below inferior nuchal line	Suboccipital n.	Extends and flexes head laterally
Obliquus capitis superior	Transverse process of atlas	Occipital bone above inferior nuchal line	Suboccipital n.	Extends, rotates, and flexes head laterally
Obliquus capitis inferior	Spine of axis	Transverse process of atlas	Suboccipital n.	Extends head and rotates it laterally
Muscles of the Neck				
Platysma	Superficial fascia over upper part of deltoid and pectoralis major	Mandible; skin and muscles over mandible and angle of mouth	Facial n.	Depresses lower jaw and lip and angle of mouth; wrinkle skin of neck
Sternocleidomastoid	Manubrium sterni and medial one-third of clavicle	Mastoid process and lateral one-half of superior nuchal line	Spinal accessory n.; C2–C3 (sensory)	Unilaterally, turns face toward opposite side; bilaterally, flexes head, raises thorax

(continued)

(continued)

Muscles	Origin	Insertion	Innervation	Action
Suprahyoid Muscles				
Digastric	Anterior belly from digastric fossa of mandible; posterior belly from mastoid notch	Intermediate tendon attached to body of hyoid	Anterior belly by mylohyoid n. of trigeminal n.; posterior belly by facial n.	Elevates hyoid and tongue; depresses mandible
Mylohyoid	Mylohyoid line of mandible	Median raphe and body of hyoid bone	Mylohyoid n. of trigeminal n.	Elevates hyoid and tongue; depresses mandible
Stylohyoid	Styloid process	Body of hyoid	Facial n.	Elevates hyoid
Geniohyoid	Genial tubercle of mandible	Body of hyoid	C1 via hypoglossal n.	Elevates hyoid and tongue
Infrahyoid Muscles				
Sternohyoid	Manubrium sterni and medial end of clavicle	Body of hyoid	Ansa cervicalis	Depresses hyoid and larynx
Sternothyroid	Manubrium sterni; first costal cartilage	Oblique line of thyroid cartilage	Ansa cervicalis	Depresses thyroid cartilage and larynx
Thyrohyoid	Oblique line of thyroid cartilage	Body and greater horn of hyoid	C1 via hypoglossal n.	Depresses and retracts hyoid and larynx

Muscles	Origin	Insertion	Innervation	Action
Omohyoid	Inferior belly from medial lip of suprascapular notch and suprascapular ligament; superior belly from intermediate tendon	Inferior belly to intermediate tendon; superior belly to body of hyoid	Ansa cervicalis	Depresses and retracts hyoid and larynx

Prevertebral Muscles

Muscles	Origin	Insertion	Innervation	Action
Anterior scalene	Transverse processes of C3–C6	Scalene tubercle on first rib	Ventral rami of cervical spinal n. (C3–C8)	Elevates first rib, bends neck
Middle scalene	Transverse processes of C2–C7	Upper surface of first rib	Ventral rami of cervical spinal n. (C3–C8)	Flexes neck laterally, elevates first rib during forced inspiration
Posterior scalene	Transverse processes of C4–C6	Outer surface of second rib	Ventral rami of cervical spinal n. (C7–C8)	Flexes neck laterally, elevates second rib during forced inspiration
Longus capitis	Transverse processes of C3–C6	Basilar part of occipital bone	Ventral rami of cervical spinal n. (C1–C4)	Flexes and rotates head

(continued)

(continued)

Muscles	Origin	Insertion	Innervation	Action
Longus colli	Transverse processes and bodies of C3–T3	Anterior tubercle of atlas; bodies of C2–C4; transverse process of C5–C6	Ventral rami of cervical spinal n. (C2–C6)	Flexes and rotates head
Rectus capitis anterior	Lateral mass of atlas	Basilar part of occipital bone	Ventral rami of cervical spinal n. (C1–C2)	Flexes and rotates head
Rectus capitis lateralis	Transverse process of atlas	Jugular process of occipital bone	Ventral rami of cervical spinal n. (C1–C2)	Flexes head laterally
Muscles of Facial Expression				
Occipitofrontalis	Superior nuchal line; upper orbital margin	Epicranial aponeurosis	Facial n.	Elevates eyebrows, wrinkles forehead
Corrugator supercilii	Medial supraorbital margin	Skin of medial eyebrow	Facial n.	Draws eyebrows downward medially
Orbicularis oculi	Medial orbital margin; medial palpebral ligament; lacrimal bone	Skin and rim of orbit; tarsal plate; lateral palpebral raphe	Facial n.	Closes eyelids
Procerus	Nasal bone and cartilage	Skin between eyebrows	Facial n.	Wrinkles skin over bones

Muscles	Origin	Insertion	Innervation	Action
Nasalis	Maxilla lateral to incisive fossa	Ala of nose	Facial n.	Draws ala of nose toward septum
Depressor septi	Incisive fossa of maxilla	Ala and nasal septum	Facial n.	Constricts nares
Orbicularis oris	Maxilla above incisor teeth	Skin of lip	Facial n.	Closes lips
Levator anguli oris	Canine fossa of maxilla	Angle of mouth	Facial n.	Elevates angle of mouth medially
Levator labii superioris	Maxilla above infraorbital foramen	Skin of upper lip	Facial n.	Elevates upper lip, dilates nares
Levator labii superioris alaeque nasi	Frontal process of maxilla	Skin of upper lip	Facial n.	Elevates ala of nose and upper lip
Zygomaticus major	Zygomatic arch	Angle of mouth	Facial n.	Draws angle of mouth backward and upward
Zygomaticus minor	Zygomatic arch	Angle of mouth	Facial n.	Elevates upper lip
Depressor labii inferioris	Mandible below mental foramen	Orbicularis oris and skin of lower lip	Facial n.	Depresses lower lip
Depressor anguli oris	Oblique line of mandible	Angle of mouth	Facial n.	Depresses angle of mouth
Risorius	Fascia over masseter	Angle of mouth	Facial n.	Retracts angle of mouth

(continued)

(continued)

Muscles	Origin	Insertion	Innervation	Action
Buccinator	Mandible; pterygomandibular raphe; alveolar processes	Angle of mouth	Facial n.	Presses cheek to keep it taut
Mentalis	Incisive fossa of mandible	Skin of chin	Facial n.	Elevates and protrudes lower lip
Auricularis anterior, superior, and posterior	Temporal fascia; epicranial aponeurosis; mastoid process	Anterior, superior, and posterior sides of auricle	Facial n.	Retract and elevate ear
Muscles of Mastication				
Temporalis	Temporal fossa	Coronoid process and ramus of mandible	Trigeminal n.	Elevates and retracts mandible
Masseter	Lower border and medial surface of zygomatic arch	Lateral surface of coronoid process, ramus and angle of mandible	Trigeminal n.	Elevates mandible
Lateral pterygoid	Superior head from infratemporal surface of sphenoid; inferior head from lateral surface of lateral pterygoid plate	Neck of mandible; articular disk and capsule of temporomandibular joint	Trigeminal n.	Protracts (protrudes) and depresses mandible

Muscles	Origin	Insertion	Innervation	Action
Medial pterygoid	Tuber of maxilla; medial surface of lateral pterygoid plate; pyramidal process of palatine bone	Medial surface of angle and ramus of mandible	Trigeminal n.	Protracts (protrudes) and elevates mandible
Muscles of Eye Movement				
Superior rectus	Common tendinous ring	Sclera just behind cornea	Oculomotor n.	Elevates eyeball
Inferior rectus	Same as above	Sclera just behind cornea	Oculomotor n.	Depresses eyeball
Medial rectus	Same as above	Sclera just behind cornea	Oculomotor n.	Adducts eyeball
Lateral rectus	Same as above	Sclera just behind cornea	Abducens n.	Adducts eyeball
Levator palpebrae superioris	Lesser wing of sphenoid above and anterior to optic canal	Tarsal plate and skin of upper eyelid	Oculomotor n.	Elevates upper eyelid
Superior oblique	Body of sphenoid bone above optic canal	Sclera beneath superior rectus	Trochlear n.	Rotates downward and medially, depresses adducted eye

(continued)

Muscles	Origin	Insertion	Innervation	Action
Inferior oblique	Floor of orbit lateral to lacrimal groove	Sclera beneath lateral rectus	Oculomotor n.	Rotates upward and laterally; elevates adducted eye
Muscles of the Palate				
Tensor veli palatini	Scaphoid fossa; spine of sphenoid; cartilage of auditory tube	Tendon hooks around hamulus of medial pterygoid plate to insert into aponeurosis of soft palate	Mandibular branch of trigeminal n.	Tenses soft palate
Levator veli palatini	Petrous part of temporal bone; cartilage of auditory tube	Aponeurosis of soft palate	Vagus n. via pharyngeal plexus	Elevates soft palate
Palatoglossus	Aponeurosis of soft palate	Dorsolateral side of tongue	Vagus n. via pharyngeal plexus	Elevates tongue
Palatopharyngeus	Aponeurosis of soft palate; hard palate	Thyroid cartilage and side of pharynx; muscles of pharynx	Vagus n. via pharyngeal plexus	Elevates pharynx; closes nasopharynx
Musculus uvulae	Posterior nasal spine of palatine bone; palatine aponeurosis	Mucous membrane of uvula	Vagus n. via pharyngeal plexus	Elevates uvula

Muscles	Origin	Insertion	Innervation	Action
Muscles of the Tongue				
Styloglossus	Styloid process	Side and inferior aspect of tongue	Hypoglossal n.	Retracts and elevates tongue
Hyoglossus	Body and greater horn of hyoid bone	Side and inferior aspect of tongue	Hypoglossal n.	Depresses and retracts tongue
Genioglossus	Genial tubercle of mandible	Inferior aspect of tongue; body of hyoid bone	Hypoglossal n.	Protrudes and depresses tongue
See Palatoglossus				
Muscles of the Pharynx				
Superior constrictor	Medial pterygoid plate; pterygoid hamulus; pterygo-mandibular raphe; mylohyoid line of mandible; side of tongue	Median raphe and pharyngeal tubercle of skull	Vagus n. via pharyngeal plexus	Constricts upper pharynx
Middle constrictor	Greater and lesser horns of hyoid; stylohyoid ligament	Median raphe	Vagus n. via pharyngeal plexus	Constricts lower pharynx
Inferior constrictor	Arch of cricoid and oblique line of thyroid cartilages	Median raphe of pharynx	Vagus n. via pharyngeal plexus, recurrent and external laryngeal n.	Constricts lower pharynx

(continued)

201

Muscles	Origin	Insertion	Innervation	Action
Stylopharyngeus	Styloid process	Thyroid cartilage and muscles of pharynx	Glossopharyngeal n.	Elevates pharynx and larynx
Salpingopharyngeus	Cartilage of auditory tube	Muscles of pharynx	Vagus n. via pharyngeal plexus	Elevates nasopharynx, opens auditory tube
See Palatopharyngeus				
Muscles of the Larynx				
Cricothyroid	Arch of cricoid cartilage	Inferior horn and lower lamina of thyroid cartilage	External laryngeal n.	Tenses vocal folds
Posterior cricoarytenoid	Posterior surface of lamina of cricoid cartilage	Muscular process of arytenoid cartilage	Recurrent laryngeal n.	Abducts vocal folds
Lateral cricoarytenoid	Arch of cricoid cartilage	Muscular process of arytenoid cartilage	Recurrent laryngeal n.	Abducts vocal folds
Transverse arytenoid	Posterior surface of arytenoid cartilage	Opposite arytenoid cartilage	Recurrent laryngeal n.	Abducts vocal folds
Oblique arytenoid	Muscular process of arytenoid cartilage	Apex of opposite arytenoid	Recurrent laryngeal n.	Abducts vocal folds
Aryepiglottic	Apex of arytenoid cartilage	Side of epiglottic cartilage	Recurrent laryngeal n.	Abducts vocal folds

Muscles	Origin	Insertion	Innervation	Action
Thyroarytenoid	Inner surface of thyroid lamina	Lateral margin of epiglottic cartilage	Recurrent laryngeal n.	Adducts vocal folds
Thyroepiglottic	Anteromedial surface of lamina of thyroid cartilage	Vocal process	Recurrent laryngeal n.	Adducts and tenses vocal folds
Vocalis	Anteromedial surface of lamina of thyroid cartilage	Anterolateral surface of arytenoid cartilage	Recurrent laryngeal n.	Adducts vocal folds
Muscles of the Middle Ear				
Stapedius	Pyramidal eminence	Neck of the stapes	Branch of the facial n.	Pulls the head of the stapes posteriorly, thereby tilting the base of the stapes and protects the inner ear from injury during a loud noise
Tensor tympani	Cartilaginous portion of the auditory tube	Handle of the malleus	Mandibular branch of trigeminal n.	Draws the manubrium medially, pulling the tympanic membrane taut

(continued)

203

(continued)

Muscles	Origin	Insertion	Innervation	Action
Muscles of the Shoulder Region				
Muscles of the Upper Limb				
Deltoid	Lateral third of clavicle, acromion, and spine of scapula	Deltoid tuberosity of humerus	Axillary n.	Anterior part: flexes and medially rotates arm; Middle part: abducts arm; Posterior part: extends and laterally rotates arm
Supraspinatus	Supraspinous fossa of scapula	Superior facet of greater tubercle of humerus	Suprascapular n.	Abducts arm
Infraspinatus	Infraspinous fossa	Middle facet of greater tubercle of humerus	Suprascapular n.	Rotates arm laterally
Subscapularis	Subscapular fossa	Lesser tubercle of humerus	Upper and lower subscapular n.	Rotates arm medially
Teres major	Dorsal surface of inferior angle of scapula	Medial lip of intertubercular groove of humerus	Lower subscapular n.	Adducts and rotates arm medially
Teres minor	Upper portion of lateral border of scapula	Lower facet of greater tubercle of humerus	Axillary n.	Rotates arm laterally

Muscles	Origin	Insertion	Innervation	Action
Latissimus dorsi	Spines of T7–T12 thoracolumbar fascia, iliac crest, ribs 9–12	Floor of bicipital groove of humerus	Thoracodorsal n.	Adducts, extends, and rotates arm medially
Muscles of the Arm				
Coracobrachialis	Coracoid process	Middle third of medial surface of humerus	Musculocutaneous n.	Flexes and adducts arm
Biceps brachii	Long head: supra-glenoid tubercle of scapula; short head: tip of coracoid process of scapula	Radial tuberosity of radius	Musculocutaneous n.	Flexes arm and forearm, supinates forearm when it is supine
Brachialis	Distal half of anterior surface of humerus	Coronoid process of ulna and ulnar tuberosity	Musculocutaneous n.	Flexes forearm
Triceps brachii	Long head: infragle-noid tubercle of scapula; Lateral head: posterior surface of humerus, superior to radial groove; Medial head: posterior surface of humerus, inferior radial groove	Posterior surface of olecranon process of ulna	Radial n.	Extends forearm

(continued)

(continued)

Muscles of the Anterior Forearm

Muscles	Origin	Insertion	Innervation	Action
Anconeus	Lateral epicondyle of humerus	Olecranon and upper posterior surface of ulna	Radial n.	Extends forearm with triceps; stabilizes elbow joint
Pronator teres	Medial epicondyle and coronoid process of ulna	Middle of lateral side of radius	Median n.	Pronates forearm
Flexor carpi radialis	Medial epicondyle of humerus	Bases of second and third metacarpals	Median n.	Flexes forearm, flexes and abducts hand
Palmaris longus	Medial epicondyle of humerus	Flexor retinaculum, palmar aponeurosis	Median n.	Flexes hand and forearm
Flexor carpi ulnaris	Medial epicondyle, medial olecranon, and posterior border of ulna	Pisiform, hook of hamate, and base of fifth metacarpal	Ulnar n.	Flexes and adducts hand, flexes forearm
Flexor digitorum superficialis	Medial epicondyle, coronoid process, oblique line of radius	Middle phalanges of finger	Median n.	Flexes proximal interphalangeal joints, flexes hand and forearm
Flexor digitorum profundus	Anteromedial surface of ulna, interosseous membrane	Bases of distal phalanges of fingers	Ulnar and median n.	Flexes distal interphalangeal joints and hand

Muscles	Origin	Insertion	Innervation	Action
Flexor pollicis longus	Anterior surface of radius, interosseous membrane, and coronoid process	Base of distal phalanx of thumb	Median n.	Flexes thumb
Pronator quadratus	Anterior surface of distal ulna	Anterior surface of distal radius	Median n.	Pronates forearm
Muscles of the Posterior Forearm				
Brachioradialis	Lateral supracondylar ridge of humerus	Base of radial styloid process	Radial n.	Flexes forearm
Extensor carpi radialis longus	Lateral supracondylar ridge of humerus	Dorsum of base of second metacarpal	Radial n.	Extends and abducts hand
Extensor carpi radialis brevis	Lateral epicondyle of humerus	Posterior base of third metacarpal	Radial n.	Extends fingers and abducts hands
Extensor digitorum	Lateral epicondyle of humerus	Extensor expansion, base of middle and digital phalanges	Radial n.	Extends fingers and hand
Extensor digiti minimi	Common extensor tendon and interosseous membrane	Extensor expansion, base of middle and distal phalanges	Radial n.	Extends little finger
Extensor carpi ulnaris	Lateral epicondyle and posterior surface of ulna	Base of fifth	Radial n.	Extends and adducts hand

(continued)

(continued)

Muscles	Origin	Insertion	Innervation	Action
Supinator	Lateral epicondyle, radial collateral and anular ligaments	Lateral side of upper part of radius	Radial n.	Supinates forearm
Abductor pollicis longus	Interosseous membrane, middle third of posterior surfaces of radius and ulna	Lateral surface of base of first metacarpal	Radial n.	Abducts thumb and hand
Extensor pollicis longus	Interosseous membrane and middle third of posterior surface of ulna	Base of distal phalanx of thumb	Radial n.	Extends distal phalanx of thumb and abducts hand
Extensor pollicis brevis	Interosseous membrane and posterior surface of middle third radius	Base of proximal phalanx of thumb	Radial n.	Extends proximal phalanx of thumb and abducts hand
Extensor indicis	Posterior surface of ulna and interosseous membrane	Extensor expansion of index finger	Radial n.	Extends index finger
Muscles of the Hand				
Abductor pollicis brevis	Flexor retinaculum, scaphoid, and trapezium	Lateral side of base of proximal phalanx of thumb	Median n.	Abducts thumb

Muscles	Origin	Insertion	Innervation	Action
Flexor pollicis brevis	Flexor retinaculum and trapezium	Base of proximal phalanx of thumb	Median n.	Flexes thumb
Opponens pollicis	Flexor retinaculum and trapezium	Lateral side of first metacarpal	Median n.	Opposes thumb to other digits
Adductor pollicis	Oblique head: capitate and bases of second and third metacarpals; Transverse head: palmar surface of third metacarpal	Medial side of base of proximal phalanx of thumb	Ulnar n.	Adducts thumb
Palmaris brevis	Medial side of flexor retinaculum, palmar aponeurosis	Skin of medial side of palm	Ulnar n.	Wrinkles skin on medial side of palm
Abductor digiti minimi	Pisiform and tendon of flexor carpi ulnaris	Medial side of base of proximal phalanx of little finger	Ulnar n.	Abducts little finger
Flexor digiti minimi brevis	Flexor retinaculum and hook of hamate	Medial side of base of proximal phalanx of little finger	Ulnar n.	Flexes proximal phalanx of little finger
Opponens digiti minimi	Flexor retinaculum and hook of hamate	Medial side of fifth metacarpal	Ulnar n.	Opposes little finger

(continued)

(continued)

Muscles	Origin	Insertion	Innervation	Action
Lumbricals (4)	Lateral side of tendons of flexor digitorum profundus	Lateral side of extensor expansion	Median (2 lateral) and ulnar (2 medial) n.	Flex metacarpophalangeal joints and extend interphalangeal joints
Dorsal interossei (4)	Adjacent sides of metacarpal bones	Lateral sides of bases of proximal phalanges; extensor expansion	Ulnar n.	Abduct fingers; flex metacarpophalangeal joints; extend interphalangeal joints
Palmar interossei (3)	Medial side of second metacarpal; lateral sides of fourth and fifth metacarpals	Bases of proximal phalanges in same sides as their origins; extensor expansion	Ulnar n.	Adduct fingers; flex metacarpophalangeal joints; extend interphalangeal joints

Appendix E
Average ROM Measurements

Shoulder

Flexion	0–180°
Extension	0–60°
Adduction/Abduction	0–180°
Horizontal Abduction	0–90°
Horizontal Adduction	0–45°
Internal Rotation	0–70°
External Rotation	0–90°
Internal Rotation (alternate method)	0–80°
External Rotation (alternate method)	0–60°

Elbow and Forearm

Extension/Flexion	0–150°
Supination	0–80°
Pronation	0–80°

Wrist

Flexion	0–80°
Extension	0–70°
Ulnar Deviation	0–30°
Radial Deviation	0–20°

Thumb

CM Flexion	0–15°
CM Extension	0–20°
MP Extension/Flexion	0–50°
IP Extension/Flexion	0–80°
Abduction	Cm
Opposition	Cm

Fingers

MP Flexion	0–90°
PIP Extension/Flexion	0–100°
DIP Extension/Flexion	0–90°
Abduction	No Norm
Adduction	No Norm

Appendix F
Prime Movers for Upper and Selected Lower Extremity Motions

Scapular elevation	Upper trapezius
	Levator scapulae
Scapular depression	Lower trapezius
	Latissimus dorsi
Scapular adduction	Middle trapezius
	Rhomboids
Scapular abduction	Serratus anterior
Shoulder flexion	Anterior deltoid
	Coracobrachialis
	Pectoralis major, clavicular head
	Biceps, both heads
Shoulder extension	Latissimus dorsi
	Teres major
	Posterior deltoid
	Triceps, long head
Shoulder abduction	Supraspinatus
	Middle deltoid
Shoulder adduction	Pectoralis major
	Teres major
	Latissimus dorsi
Shoulder horizontal abduction	Posterior deltoid
Shoulder horizontal adduction	Pectoralis major
	Anterior deltoid
Shoulder external rotation	Infraspinatus
	Teres minor
	Posterior deltoid
Shoulder internal rotation	Subscapularis
	Teres major
	Latissimus dorsi
	Pectoralis major
	Anterior deltoid
Elbow flexion	Biceps
	Brachialis
	Brachioradialis
Elbow extension	Triceps
Pronation	Pronator teres
	Pronator quadratus

Supination	Supinator
	Biceps
Wrist extension	Extensor carpi radialis longus (ECRL)
	Extensor carpi radialis brevis (ECRB)
	Extensor carpi ulnaris (ECU)
Wrist flexion	Flexor carpi radialis (FCR)
	Palmaris longus
	Flexor carpi ulnaris (FCU)
Finger DIP flexion	Flexor digitorum profundus (FDP)
Finger PIP flexion	Flexor digitorum superficialis (FDS)
	Flexor digitorum profundus (FDP)
Finger MP flexion	Flexor digitorum profundus (FDP)
	Flexor digitorum superficialis (FDS)
	Dorsal interossei
	Volar (palmar) interossei
	Flexor digiti minimi (small finger only)
Finger adduction	Volar (palmar) interossei
Finger abduction	Dorsal interossei
	Abductor digiti minimi (small finger only)
Finger MP extension	Extensor digitorum (ED)
	Extensor indicis proprius (index finger only)
	Extensor digiti minimi (small finger only)
Finger PIP/DIP extension	Lumbricales
	Dorsal and volar (palmar) interossei
	Extensor digitorum (ED)
	Extensor indicis proprius (index finger only)
	Extensor digiti minimi (small finger only)
Thumb IP extension	Extensor pollicis longus (EPL)

213

Thumb MP extension	Extensor pollicis brevis (EPB)
	Extensor pollicis longus (EPL)
Thumb abduction	Abductor pollicis longus (APL)
	Abductor pollicis brevis (APB)
Thumb IP flexion	Flexor pollicis longus (FPL)
Thumb MP flexion	Flexor pollicis brevis (FPB)
	Flexor pollicis longus (FPL)
Thumb adduction	Adductor pollicis
Opposition	Opponens pollicis (thumb)
	Opponens digiti minimi (small finger)
Hip flexion	Iliopsoas—Iliacus and psoas major
Hip extension	Gluteus maximus
	Biceps femoris
Knee flexion	Semimembranosus
	Semitendinosus
	Biceps femoris
Knee extension	Rectus femoris
	Vastus medialis
	Vastus intermedius
	Vastus lateralis
Ankle dorsiflexion	Tibialis anterior
	Extensor hallucis longus
	Extensor digitorum longus
Ankle plantar flexion	Gastrocnemius
	Soleus

Appendix G
Web Resources

Athletic Injuries
American College of Sports Medicine: http://www.acsm.org

American Sports Medicine Institute: http://www.asmi.org

Institute for Preventative Sports Medicine: http://www.ipsm.org

International Federation of Sports Medicine: http://www.fims.org

The Physician and Sportsmedicine Online:
  http://www.physsportsmed.com

Attention Deficit and Hyperactivity Disorder
KidSource Online: http://www.kidsource.com/kidsource/
  content2/add.nimh.html

National Institute of Mental Health: http://www.nimh.nih.gov/
  publicat/adhd.cfm

National Library of Medicine: http://www.nlm.nih.gov/pubs/
  cbm/adhd.html

Optometrists Network: http://www.add-adhd.org

Autism
Autism Research Institute:
  http://www.autism.com/ari/contents.html

The Autism Society of America: http://www.autism-society.org

Center for the Study of Autism: http://www.autism.org

National Alliance for Autism Research: http://www.naar.org

National Institute of Mental Health: http://www.nimh.nih.gov/
  publicat/autism.cfm

Brachial Plexus Injury
Brachial Plexus Palsy Foundation: http://membrane.com/bpp/
  protocol.html

Texas Children's Hospital, Department of Pediatric Neurosurgery:
  http://www.bcm.tmc.edu/pednsurg/disorder/brachial.htm

United Brachial Plexus Network: http://www.ubpn.org

Cardiac Dysfunction
American Heart Association: http://www.americanheart.org

American Heart Lung and Blood Institute: http://www.nhlbi.nih.gov

U.K. Department of Health, National Service Framework for Coronary Heart Disease: http://www.doh.gov.uk/nsf/coronary.htm

Carpal Tunnel Syndrome

ald.net Services: http://www.carpal-tunnel.com

American Hand Therapy Foundation: http://www.ahtf.org

American Society of Hand Therapists: http://www.asht.org

University of Washington Orthopaedics and Sports Medicine: http://www.orthop.washington.edu/hand_wrist/carpaltunnel/01

Cerebral Palsy

American Academy for Cerebral Palsy and Developmental Medicine: http://www.aacpdm.org

Cerebral Palsy Association in Canada: http://www.cerebralpalsycanada.com

National Institute of Neurological Disorders and Stroke: http://www.ninds.nih.gov/health_and_medical/disorders/cerebral_palsy.htm

United Cerebral Palsy: http://www.ucpa.org

Depression

Depression and Bipolar Support Alliance (formerly the National Depressive and Manic-Depressive Association): http://www.ndmda.org

Depression and Related Affective Disorders Association: http://www.drada.org

National Alliance for Research on Schizophrenia and Depression: http://www.narsad.org

National Institute of Mental Health: http://www.nimh.nih.gov/publicat/depressionmenu.cfm

Diabetes Mellitus

American Diabetes Association: http://www.diabetes.org

Diabetes UK: http://www.diabetes.org.uk

Mayfield, J. (1998, October 15). "Diagnosis and classification of diabetes mellitus: New criteria," *American Family Physician*, p. 1355 [On-line]. Available: http://www.aafp.org/afp/981015ap/mayfield.html

The National Diabetes Center: http://www.diabetes-mellitus.org

Guillain-Barré Syndrome

Disability Resources.org:
  http://www.disabilityresources.org/GB.html
Guillain-Barré Syndrome Foundation International:
  http://www.guillain-barre.com

Hand Injuries

American Hand Therapy Foundation: http://www.ahtf.org

American Occupational Therapy Association: http://www.aota.org

American Physical Therapy Association: http://www.apta.org

American Society of Hand Therapists: http://www.asht.org

Canadian Society of Hand Therapists: http://www.csht.org

HIV/AIDS

American Society for Clinical Pathology: http://www.ascp.org/
  general/pub_resources/aids
HIV/AIDS Treatment Information Service, U.S. Department of Health
  and Human Services: http://www.hivatis.org
Johns Hopkins AIDS Service: http://www.hopkins-aids.edu
Journal of the American Medical Association HIV/AIDS Resource
  Center: http://www.ama-assn.org/special/hiv/hivhome.htm

Homelessness

Institute for the Study of Homelessness and Poverty:
  http://www.weingart.org
National Alliance to End Homelessness: http://www.naeh.org
National Law Center on Homelessness and Poverty:
  http://www.nlchp.org
National Resource Center on Homelessness and Mental Illness:
  http://www.nrchmi.com
U.S. Department of Health and Human Services:
  http://aspe.hhs.gov/progsys/homeless

Learning Disability

British Institute of Learning Disabilities: http://www.bild.org.uk

LD Resources: http://www.ldresources.com

Learning Disabilities Association of America: http://www.ldanatl.org

Learning Disabilities Association of Canada: http://www.ldac-taac.ca

Low Back Pain

Bratton, R. L. (1999, November 15). "Assessment and management of acute low back pain." *American Family Physician*, p. 2299 [Online]. Available: http://www.aafp.org/afp/991115ap/2299.html.

Non-Surgical Orthopaedic and Spine Center:
http://www.lowbackpain.com

Lymphedema

Circle of Hope Lymphedema Foundation:
http://www.lymphedemacircleofhope.org

Lymphedema Awareness Foundation: http://www.lymphaware.org

National Lymphedema Network: http://www.lymphnet.org

Multiple Sclerosis

Multiple Sclerosis Association of America: http://www.msaa.com

Multiple Sclerosis Foundation: http://www.msfacts.org

Multiple Sclerosis Society of Canada: http://www.mssociety.ca

National Multiple Sclerosis Society: http://www.nmss.org

Muscular Dystrophy

DMD Forum: http://www.dmdforum.org

Muscular Dystrophy Association: http://www.mdausa.org

Society for Muscular Dystrophy Information International:
http://www.nsnet.org/smdi

Myasthenia Gravis

MEDLINE Plus Health Information: http://www.nlm.nih.gov/
medlineplus/myastheniagravis.html

Myasthenia Gravis Foundation of America:
http://www.myasthenia.org

National Institute of Neurological Disorders and Stroke:
http://www.ninds.nih.gov/health_and_medical/disorders/
myasthenia_gravis.htm

Personality Disorder

Borderline Personality Disorder Research Foundation:
http://www.borderlineresearch.org

Borderline Personality Disorder Central:
http://www.bpdcentral.com

National Institute of Mental Health: http://www.nimh.nih.gov/
publicat/bpd.cfm

Mental Help Net: http://mentalhelp.net/poc/center_index.php?id=8

Post Polio Syndrome

Easter Seals Colorado: http://www.eastersealsco.org/postpolio/postpolio.html

National Institute of Neurological Disorders and Stroke: http://www.ninds.nih.gov/health_and_medical/disorders/post_polio_short.htm

Post Traumatic Stress Disorder

American Psychiatric Association: http://www.psych.org/public_info/ptsd.cfm

Madison Institute of Medicine, Facts for Health: http://ptsd.factsforhealth.org

National Center for Posttraumatic Stress Disorder: http://www.ncptsd.org

Posttraumatic Stress Disorder Alliance: http://www.ptsdalliance.org

Rheumatoid Arthritis

American College of Rheumatology: http://www.rheumatology.org

Arthritis Care: http://www.arthritiscare.org.uk

Arthritis Foundation: http://www.arthritis.org

Arthritis Research: http://arthritis-research.com

MedicineNet: http://www.focusonarthritis.com

National Institute of Arthritis and Musculoskeletal and Skin Diseases: http://www.niams.nih.gov

Sensory Integration Dysfunction

Children's Disabilities Information: http://www.childrensdisabilities.info/sensory_integration

Sensory Integration Network: http://www.sinetwork.org

Spinal Cord Injury

Foundation for Spinal Cord Injury Prevention, Care & Cure: http://www.fscip.org

National Spinal Cord Injury Association: http://www.spinalcord.org

Spinal Cord Injury Network International: http://www.spinalcordinjury.org

Spinal Cord Injury Resource Center: http://www.spinalinjury.net

Stroke

American Stroke Association: http://www.strokeassociation.org

Heart and Stroke Foundation of Canada: http://ww2.heartandstroke.ca

National Institute of Neurological Disorders and Stroke: http://www.ninds.nih.gov/health_and_medical/disorders/stroke.htm

National Stroke Association: http://www.stroke.org

Glossary

activities of daily living (ADL): self-maintenance tasks considered necessary for maintaining the demands of daily living including such activities as grooming, bathing, dressing, toileting and personal hygiene, taking medication, and self-feeding

acute: very severe or sharp, as in pain; disease or symptoms with rapid, severe onset

adapt: change task or environment demands to support performance

adaptation: making the tasks simpler or less physically demanding to promote functional independence; changing in response to new demands or expectations

adult day care: programs that last several hours a day and provide meaningful, structured activities to assist people with physical, emotional, or cognitive disabilities to remain living at home, and to provide respite for primary caregivers

affect: the emotional tone of an individual demonstrated by facial expressions and vocal inflection

agnosia: inability to recognize familiar objects in spite of intact sensory capacities

alcoholism: a chronic illness characterized by extreme dependence on alcohol and corresponding disturbances in the individual's family, social, and work life

Americans with Disabilities Act (ADA): a civil rights act that provides protection to individuals with disabilities in the workplace

amputation: surgical or traumatic removal of a part of the body, typically all or part of a limb; may also be a congenital defect

amyotrophic lateral sclerosis (ALS): a degenerative disease that destroys motor neurons in the cortex, brainstem, and spinal cord, leading to weakness, muscle atrophy, and death

anorexia nervosa: self-induced starvation, often a chronic condition with medical and psychological components

aphasia: impairment of language; receptive aphasia—the inability to understand written or spoken language; expressive aphasia—impairment in the use of verbal and written language

apraxia: inability to perform motor activities although sensory motor function is intact and the individual understands the requirements of the task

arthritis: a common chronic condition of the joints that results in pain, loss of motion, deformity, and associated functional deficits

arthroplasty: surgical intervention to reconstruct or replace a damaged joint

assessment: specific tools or instruments used as part of the evaluation process

assessment of motor and process skills (AMPS): assessment used to examine the relationship between motor and process skills and task performance, to determine current level of task competence, and to predict performance in IADL

assistive technology device: a piece of equipment or product acquired off-the-shelf, modified or customized and used to improve or maintain functional capabilities of an individual with a disability

attention: the cognitive ability to focus on a task, issue, or object

attention deficit/hyperactive disorder (ADHD): a disorder characterized by inattention or attention deficit, overactivity, and impulsiveness

autism: a pervasive developmental disorder characterized by deficits in social interaction, communication; people with autism demonstrate restrictive and repetitive behavior

bilateral integration: using both sides of the body in a coordinated manner during activity

bipolar disorder: also called manic depression; characterized by cycles of mania and depression persisting for at least a week or severe enough for hospitalization

bradycardia: abnormally slow heart rate, with a pulse rate less than 60 beats per minute

bradypnea: a slow respiratory rate

bulimia nervosa: eating disorder consisting of binge eating followed by self-induced vomiting, or use of laxatives; excessive exercising or fasting to compensate for the binging

Canadian Occupational Performance Measure (COPM): client-centered, semi-structured interview procedure designed to measure a client's perceptions of his or her occupational performance over time

cerebral palsy: condition caused by damage to the brain, usually occurring before, during, or shortly after birth, with associated impairments that may include: visual and auditory deficits, seizures, mental retardation, learning disabilities, oral motor and behavioral problems

cerebrovascular accident (CVA): also called stroke or "brain-attack," characterized by an interruption in blood supply that causes injury to the brain resulting in neurological deficits in a specific area

chronic illness: illness of long duration, showing little change or with slow progression that can lead to decline in functional ability

chronic obstructive pulmonary disorder (COPD): a variety of pulmonary disorders including: chronic bronchitis, asthma, emphysema, and bronchiectasis; implies irreversible airway damage

chronic pain: pain, often less intense than acute pain, which continues and recurs over a long period of time

cognition: ability to think and reason to solve problems

concept: construct or idea

contracture: decrease in length of soft tissue that can lead to decreased joint motion

coordination—fine: smooth patterns of movement, typically of the upper extremity, such as those required for buttoning, typing, writing

coordination—gross: smooth patterns of movement, particularly of large muscle groups, such as those required for walking, lifting, and running

dementias: mental states with symptoms of memory impairment and abstract thinking that are severe enough to impair function in an individual who was previously unimpaired

depression: a mood disorder characterized by extreme sadness, feelings of hopelessness, worthlessness, and dejection that are pervasive and interfere with daily activities of living

developmental delay: a deficit in one or more of the following areas of development: cognitive, physical, communication, social or emotional, and adaptive or self-help skills

developmental disabilities: a group of chronic conditions including mental retardation, cerebral palsy, genetic and chromosomal anomalies, autism, learning disabilities, severe orthopedic impairments, visual and hearing deficits, serious emotional disturbances, and traumatic brain injury

Diagnostic and Statistical Manual of Mental Disorders, 4th Edition *(DSM-IV):* guide for the diagnosis of psychiatric conditions; includes diagnostic criteria, symptoms, prevalence, and course of the disease or condition

emphysema: enlargement of the airspaces distal to the terminal nonrespiratory bronchioles, accompanied by destructive changes of the alveolar walls

endurance: the ability to continue an activity over time

environment: physical (geography, objects, living spaces) and social (people, culture, familial)

evaluation: an information-gathering event to identify problems being experienced by a person initially, during, and upon discharge; may include observation, interview, or use of standardized and nonstandardized assessment tools

family-centered care: care implemented and provided through the combined efforts of family members and practitioners

Functional Independence Measure (FIM^{SM}): a measure of functional status that reflects the impact of disability on the individual and on the human and economic resources of the community

generalization: the spontaneous ability to transfer what is learned in one situation to a different situation

Guillain-Barré syndrome: a peripheral nerve disorder characterized by an acute inflammation of multiple nerves, leading to development of rapid muscular weakness, potential paralysis, and sensory impairment or loss

hemianopsia: blindness in half of the field of vision in one or both eyes

hypertonia: high muscle tone that results in slow, difficult movements, requiring excessive efforts

hypertrophic scar: excessive scar formation that rises above the level of the skin plane but does not extend beyond the original borders of the burn wound

hypotension (low blood pressure): blood pressure consistently less than 90/60 mmHg

hypotonia: low muscle tone that interferes with the balance between stability and mobility required for almost all movement, especially movement against gravity

Individual Education Plan (IEP): a plan developed and coordinated by the school placement team to support the learning of a child with a disability that has an effect on school performance

instrumental activities of daily living (IADL): activities such as menu planning, budgeting, shopping, food preparation, medication management, and community access

interdisciplinary team: a type of team in which members share responsibility for providing services; team members carry out separate evaluations, sharing the results in order to develop an integrated care plan

interview: a communication process between interviewer and interviewee involving questions and answers; a shared process of discovery

joint protection: techniques designed to minimize stress to joints damaged by arthritis or other musculoskeletal conditions

Kohlman Evaluation of Living Skills (KELS): standardized assessment designed to aid in discharge planning for clients with psychiatric or cognitive diagnoses by evaluating the ability to live independently and safely in the community

learning disability: a chronic condition of neurological origin that interferes with the development, integration, and use of verbal and nonverbal abilities

leisure: activities driven by internal motivation (free will), not usually done within time constraints

measurement: process of assigning numbers to represent quantities of a trait, attribute, or characteristic; to quantify aspects of people, but not people themselves

Medicaid: a health insurance program for the poor paid for with federal funds requiring state matching funds

Medicare: a federal health insurance program administered by the Social Security Administration and the Centers for Medicare and Medicaid Services

memory: the ability to register, retain, and recall past experiences, knowledge, or sensations

mental retardation: general term used to describe a lifelong developmental disability marked by intellectual and functional skills deficits

Mini-Mental State Examination (MMSE): a standardized assessment developed as a short and simple quantitative measure of cognitive performance in the neurogeriatric population, intended for clinical use in routine and serial examinations of mental status

motor learning: acquiring and modifying motor behavior

motor planning: the ability to carry out a skilled, nonhabitual motor activity

multiple sclerosis (MS): progressive disease characterized by a demyelinization or destruction of the myelin sheath that covers the nerve fibers within the central nervous system (brain and spinal cord)

muscle strength: the ability to produce movement or to resist an external force

muscle tone: resistance to stretch or mild contraction of muscle at rest

muscular dystrophy: a group of genetically determined, painless, degenerative myopathies that are progressively debilitating as muscles gradually weaken and atrophy

myasthenia gravis (MG): progressive, degenerative muscle disease that occurs at the site of the myoneural junction, resulting in weakness from the decrease in the numbers of receptors for neurotransmitters

neoplasm: abnormal proliferation of cells as a tumor or growth

neural tube defect: spina bifida; spine is cleft or split because the vertebrae do not enclose the spinal cord during the first trimester of pregnancy, resulting in abnormal development of the meninges, nerves, and vertebrae

occupation: the daily activities typical for a culture that form a pattern of activity

occupational role: behavioral expectations that fit with an individual's position or status in the social system

orientation: awareness of self in relation to time, place, and identification of others

orthopedics: related to the dysfunction of bones, joints, and their related structures: muscles, tendons, ligaments, and nerves

orthotics: the designing, fabrication, and fitting of orthopedic appliances

osteoarthritis: a progressive, degenerative joint disease affecting the joints of the fingers, elbows, hips, knees, and ankles; results in limitations of movement and deterioration of joint articular surfaces

pain: discomfort caused by noxious stimulation of sensory nerve endings; pain is a subjective and varies from one person to the next; can be an important diagnostic symptom

paralysis: loss or impairment of motor or sensory function of body part caused by injury to central or peripheral nervous system tissue

Parkinson's disease: neurological symptom complex characterized by rigidity, tremor, akinesia, and loss of spontaneous and automatic movement

perception: mental process by which intellectual, sensory, and emotional data are organized meaningfully; conscious recognition and interpretation of sensory stimuli

performance areas: activities of daily living, work and productive activity, and play and leisure activities

performance components: skills used to engage in daily activities: sensory processing, perceptual processing, neuromusculoskeletal, motor, cognitive integration, and psychosocial skills/psychological components

phantom limb pain: pain that is perceived to be in the amputated limb

physical environment: nonhuman aspects of the environment, including landscape, buildings, furniture, tools, and implements

play and leisure activities: intrinsically motivating activities that provide pleasure, relaxation, and the ability to express oneself creatively

psychometrics: the process by which psychological and intelligence tests are developed, administered, and interpreted

range of motion (ROM): the arc through which a joint moves; can be measured actively (AROM), passively (PROM), or both

reliability: a characteristic of a test or measurement in which the same results occur with repeated trials; the measure is consistent

rheumatoid arthritis (RA): a progressive systemic disease characterized by remissions and exacerbations of destructive inflammation of connective tissue, results in limitations in range of motion and deformity

roles: give people scripts to behave in ways consistent with their social roles, examples being student, worker, parent, and clergy

schizophrenia: a group of related psychotic disorders that produce disturbed thought processes, leading to difficulties of communication, interpersonal relationships, and reality testing

scoliosis: lateral curvature of the spine

screening: a cursory evaluation, generally not requested by a physician, done to determine if a more intensive evaluation is indicated

self-care: activities that individuals engage in on their own behalf to maintain their health and well-being, such as eating, bathing, grooming, and personal hygiene

self-report measures: surveys, forms, and checklists that the client completes on his or her own

sensation: the transmission to the brain of nerve impulses caused by stimulation of a sensory receptor site, resulting in awareness of this stimulation

sensory integration: the organization of sensation to form perceptions, behaviors, and to learn; a neurological process and a theory of the relationship between the neural organization of sensory processing and behavior

spasticity: excessive tone in a muscle typically caused by an upper motor neuron lesion

spina bifida: See *neural tube defect*

spinal cord injury: any traumatic event that causes damage to the spinal cord leading to loss (complete or partial) of function below the level of injury

standardized tests: instruments that have established and tested norms

static splint: splint or orthotic device with no moving parts; maintains a joint or joints in desired position

stereognosis: perception and identification of the form and nature of an object through the sense of touch

subluxation: incomplete or partial dislocation of a joint; commonly noted in the shoulder, wrist, and fingers

substance abuse: impairment secondary to the use of drugs, alcohol, or other substance

tactile: pertaining to touch

tactile localization: ability to determine the location of a cutaneous stimulus

total hip replacement (THR): surgical removal of the head of the femur and the acetabulum and replacement with metal and plastic components

traumatic brain injury (TBI): damage to the brain as a result of an external force such as in a car accident, fall, gunshot wound, or other trauma

uniform terminology: a standard terminology developed by the American Occupational Therapy Association to facilitate use of consistent language for documentation, reimbursement, management, and research

unilateral inattention: also called unilateral neglect, the lack of awareness of stimuli presented to the side opposite the cerebral lesion in individuals who do not have primary sensory or motor impairments

upper motor neuron lesions: area of injury with the central nervous system (cortex and spinal cord) resulting in loss of voluntary muscle control and a loss of inhibition on reflexive movement causing hyperreflexia

validity: a psychometric property that is concerned with the capacity of the measurement instrument to measure what is supposed to be measured

vestibular system: structures of the inner ear associated with balance and position sense

visual accommodation: ability to focus on an object at varying distances

visual perception: cognitive process of obtaining and interpreting visual information from the environment; includes discrimination, memory, spatial relationships, form constancy, sequential memory, figure-ground, and closure

Suggested Reading

Amyotrophic Lateral Sclerosis Association. (n.d.). *Research*. Retrieved December 11, 2002, from http://www.alsa.org/research.

Brazelton, T. B. (1984). *Neonatal behavioral assessment scale* (2nd ed.). Philadelphia: Lippincott.

Coppard, B. M., & Lohman, H. (2001). *Introduction to splinting: A critical-reasoning and problem-solving approach* (2nd ed.). St. Louis, MO: Mosby.

Dean, E. (1994). Cardiac development. In B. R. Bonder & M. B. Wagner (Eds.), *Functional performance in older adults*. Philadelphia: F. A. Davis.

Engstrom, B., & Van de Ven, C. (1999). *Therapy for amputees* (3rd ed.). London: Churchill Livingstone.

Gallo, J. J., Busby-Whitehead, J., Rabins, P. V., Silliman, R. A., & Murphy, J. B. (1999). *Reichel's care of the elderly: Clinical aspects of aging* (5th ed.). Philadelphia: Lippincott, Williams & Wilkins.

Grabowski, J. (1984). Cocaine: Introduction and overview. In J. Grabowski (Ed.), *Cocaine: Pharmacology, effects, and treatment of abuse*. Washington, DC: NIDA Research Monograph Series 50, 1–8.

Horn, L. J., & Zasler, N. D. (1996). *Medical rehabilitation of traumatic brain injury*. St. Louis, MO: Mosby.

International Association of the Study of Pain. (n.d.). *Website*. Retrieved December 10, 2002, from http:www.iasp-pain.org.

Johnson, M. (1977). Assessment of clinical pain. In A. K. Jacox (Ed.), *Pain: A source book for nurses and other health professionals* (pp. 139–166). Boston: Little, Brown & Co.

MacGregor, S. N., Keith, L. G., & Chasnoff, I. J., et al. (1987). Cocaine use during pregnancy: Adverse perinatal outcome. *American Journal of Obstetrics and Gynecology, 157*, 686–690.

Malkmus, D., Booth, B. J., & Kodimer, C. (1980). *Rehabilitation of the head-injured adult: Comprehensive cognitive management*. Downey, CA: Professional Staff Association of Rancho Los Amigos Hospital.

Muller, M. J., et al. (1994). Modern treatment of a burn wound. In R. L. Richard & M. J. Staley (Eds.), *Burn care and rehabilitation: Principles and practice.* Philadelphia: F. A. Davis.

National Institute on Aging. (1996). *Progress report on Alzheimer's disease, 1996* (NIH Publication No. 96-4137). Washington, DC: National Institutes of Health.

Platt, J. (1996). *Occupational therapy practice guidelines for adults with hip fractures/replacement.* Bethesda, MD: American Occupational Therapy Association.

Polygenis, D., et al. (1998). Moderate alcohol consumption during pregnancy and the incidence of fetal malformations: A meta-analysis. *Neurotoxicology and Teratology, 20,* 61–67.

Ponchillia, P., & Ponchillia, S. (Eds.) (1996). *Foundations of rehabilitation teaching with persons who are blind or visually impaired.* New York: American Foundation for the Blind Press.

Psychologynet. (2002). *Online psychological services: Posttraumatic stress disorder.* Retrieved December 10, 2002, from http://www.psychologynet.org/ptsd.html.

Punwar, A. J., & Peloquin, S. M. (2000). *Occupational therapy: Principles and practice* (3rd ed.). Philadelphia: Lippincott, Williams & Wilkins.

Stein, F., & Cutler, S. (2002). *Psychosocial occupational therapy: A holistic approach* (2nd ed.). Clifton Park, NY: Delmar Learning.

Streissguth, A., & Kanter, J. (1997). *The challenge of fetal alcohol syndrome.* Seattle, WA: University of Washington.

References

Adler, C. (1996). Spinal cord injury. In L. W. Pedretti (Ed.), *Occupational therapy: Practice skills for physical dysfunction* (4th ed.). Chicago: Mosby.

American Heart Association. (1979). *The exercise standards book.* Dallas, TX: Author.

American Psychiatric Association. (1994). *Diagnostic and statistical manual of mental disorders* (4th ed.). Washington, DC: Author.

American Psychiatric Association. (2000). *Diagnostic and statistical manual of mental disorders* (4th ed. text revision). Washington, DC: Author.

Antonarakis, S. E., & Down Syndrome Collaborative Group. (1991). Parental origin of the extra chromosome in trisomy 21 as indicated by analysis of DNA polymorphisms. *New England Journal of Medicine, 324,* 872–876.

Arkwright, N. (1998). *An introduction to sensory integration.* San Antonio, TX: Therapy Skill Builders.

Arthritis Foundation. (2001). *Primer on the rheumatic diseases* (12th ed.). Atlanta, GA: Author.

Ayres, J. (1972). *Sensory integration and learning disorders.* Los Angeles, CA: Western Psychological Services.

Bachelder, J. (1994). Rehabilitation. In B. Bonder & M. Wagner (Eds.), *Functional performance in older adults* (pp. 86–108). Philadelphia: F.A. Davis.

Beers, M. H., & Berkow, R. (1999). *The Merck manual of diagnosis and therapy* (17th ed.). Whitehouse Station, NJ: Merck Research Laboratories.

Belcher, J. R., Scholler-Jacquish, A., & Drummond, M. (1991). Three stages of homelessness: A conceptual model for social work in healthcare. *Health Social Work, 16*(2), 87–93.

Biederman, J., & Faraone, S. (1996). Attention deficit hyperactivity disorder. *On the Brain: The Harvard Mahoney Neuroscience Institute Newsletter, 5*(1). Retrieved October 1, 2002, from http://www.med.harvard.edu/publications/On_The_Brain/Volume5/Number1/ADD.html.

Brigham, P.A., & McLoughlin, E. (1996). Burn incidence and medical care use in the United States: Estimates, trends, and data sources. *Journal of Burn Care and Rehabilitation, 17,* 95–107.

Brummel-Smith, K. (1990). Rehabilitation. In C. K. Cassel, R. M. Leipzig, H. J. Cohen, E. B. Larson, D. E. Meier, & C. F. Capello (Eds.), *Geriatric medicine* (pp. 214-234). New York: Springer-Verlag.

Burke, D. T., Burke, M. M., Stewart, G. W., & Cambre, A. (1994). Splinting for carpal tunnel syndrome: In search of the optimal angle. *Archives of Physical Medicine and Rehabilitation, 75*(11), 1241-1244.

Buschbacher, L. (1996). *Rehabilitation of patients with peripheral neuropathies.* Philadelphia: W. B. Saunders.

Cammisa, K. M., & Hobbs, S. G. (1993). Etiology of autism: A review of recent biogenic theories and research. *Occupational Therapy in Mental Health, 12*(2), 39-67.

CHADD: Children and Adults with Attention-Deficit/Hyperactivity Disorder. (2001). *The disorder named AD/HD* (CHADD Fact Sheet 1). Retrieved December 10, 2002, from http://www.chadd.org/fs/fs1.htm.

Cummings, S. R., Kelsey, J. L., Nevitt, M. C., & O'Dowd, K. J. (1985). Epidemiology of osteoporosis and osteoporotic fractures. *Epidemiological Review, 7,* 178-208.

Davis, L., & Kirkland, M. (1988). *Role of occupational therapy with the elderly.* Rockville, MD: American Occupational Therapy Association.

Dean, E., & Ross, J. (1992). Oxygen transport: The basis for contemporary cardiopulmonary physical therapy and its optimization with body positioning and mobilization. *Physical Therapy Practice, 4*(1), 34-44.

Developmental Disabilities Assistance and Bill of Rights Amendments of 1987, Pub. L. No. 100-146, 42 U.S.C. Sec. 6000 (1989).

Duran, L., & Fisher, A. G. (1999). Evaluation and intervention with executive functions impairment. In C. Unsworth (Ed.), *Cognitive and perceptual dysfunction: A clinical reasoning approach to evaluation and intervention* (pp. 209-255). Philadelphia: F. A. Davis.

Frankel, D. (1995). Multiple sclerosis. In D. A. Umphred (Ed.), *Neurological rehabilitation* (pp. 588-605). St. Louis, MO: Mosby.

Friedman, M. J. (2002, October 13). *Posttraumatic stress disorder: An overview.* Retrieved December 10, 2002, from http://www.ncptsd.org/facts/general/fs_overview.html.

Gillen, G., & Burkhardt, A. (1998). *Stroke rehabilitation: A function-based approach*. St. Louis, MO: Mosby.

Gower, D., & Bowker, M. (1993). The elderly with hip arthroplasty. In S. E. Ryan (Ed.), *Practice issues in occupational therapy: Intraprofessional team building* (pp. 161-168). Thorofare, NJ: Slack.

Harrow, M., Sands, J. R., Silverstein, M. L., & Goldberg, J. F. (1997). Course and outcome for schizophrenia versus other psychotic patients: A longitudinal study. *Schizophrenia Bulletin, 23,* 287-302.

Hayes, A., & Batshaw, M. L. (1993). *Clinics of North America, 40,* 523-535.

Hollar, L. D. (1995). Spinal cord injury. In C. A. Trombly (Ed.), *Occupational therapy for physical dysfunction* (4th ed., pp. 795-813). Baltimore: Williams & Wilkins.

Individuals with Disabilities Education Act of 1990, 20 U.S.C. Sec. 1400 *et seq.*

Jennett, B., & Teasdale, G. (1981). *Management of head injuries*. Philadelphia: F. A. Davis.

Jose, R. T. (Ed.). (1983). *Understanding low vision*. New York: American Foundation for the Blind.

Kasch, M. C. (1996). Hand injuries. In L. W. Pedretti (Ed.), *Occupational therapy: Practice skills for physical dysfunction* (4th ed.). Chicago: Mosby.

Katz, D. J. (1992). Neuropathology and neurobehavioral recovery from closed head injury. *Journal of Head Trauma Rehabilitation, 7,* 1-15.

Kautzmann, L. (1984). *Occupational therapy in health care, 1*(2), 45-52.

Larson, B. A. (1996). *Occupational therapy practice guidelines for adults with low back pain*. Bethesda, MD: American Occupational Therapy Association.

Laskowski, E. R. (1996). Concepts in sports medicine. In R. L. Braddom, R. M. Buschbacher, D. Dumitru, E. W. Johnson, D. J. Matthews, & M. Sinaki (Eds.), *Physical medicine and rehabilitation*. Philadelphia: W. B. Saunders.

Lewis, C., & Bottomley, J. (1996). Musculoskeletal changes with age: Clinical implications. In C. Lewis (Ed.), *Aging: Health care's challenge* (3rd ed., pp. 147-174). Philadelphia: F. A. Davis.

MacRae, A., & Riley, E. (1990). Home health occupational therapy for the management of chronic pain: An environmental model. *Occupational Therapy Practice, 1*(3), 69-76.

Magaziner J., Simonsick, E. M., Kashner, M., Hebel, J. R., & Kenzora, J. E. (1990). Predictors of functional recovery one year following hospital discharge for hip fracture: A prospective study. *Journal of Gerontology, 45,* M101-107.

Mayfield, J. (1998). *Diagnosis and classification of diabetes mellitus: New criteria.* Retrieved October 2, 2002, from http://www.aafp.org/afp/981015ap/mayfield.html.

Mayo Clinic. (2001). *Post-traumatic stress disorder.* Retrieved December 10, 2002, from http://www.mayoclinic.com/findinformation/diseasesandconditions/invoke.cfm?id=DS00246.

McCormack, G. L., & Pedretti, L. W. (1996). Motor unit dysfunction. In L. W. Pedretti (Ed.), *Occupational therapy: Practice skills for physical dysfunction* (4th ed., pp. 756-757). St. Louis: Mosby.

Mental Retardation Facilities and Community Health Centers Act, Pub. L. 88-164 (1963).

Mersky, H. (1986). Classification of chronic pain: Description of chronic pain syndromes and definition of pain terms. *Pain (Suppl. 3),* S217.

Morris, P. A., & Muhn, L. (1998). Amputation and prosthetics. In M. B. Early (Ed.), *Physical dysfunction practice skills for the occupational therapy assistant* (pp. 456-468). St. Louis, MO: Mosby.

Muscular Dystrophy Association. (2001). *Limb-girdle muscular dystrophy.* Retrieved December 10, 2002, from http://www.mdusa.org/disease/lgmd.html.

Mutran, E. J., Reitzes, D. C., Mossey, J., Fernandez, J., & Erlinda, M. (1998). Social support, depression and recovery of walking ability following hip fracture surgery. *Journal of Gerontology, 50B,* S354-S361.

National Center for Learning Disabilities. (1999). *About LD: LD Basics.* Retrieved December 10, 2002, from http://www.ncld.org/info.

National CJD Surveillance Unit. (2001). *Creutzfeldt-Jakob Disease Surveillance in the UK: Tenth Annual Report.* Retrieved December 10, 2002, from http://www.cjd.ed.ac.uk/rep2001.html.

National Institute of Mental Health. (1999). *Schizophrenia* (NIH Publication No. 99-3517). Retrieved December 11, 2002, from http://www.nimh.nih.gov/publicat/schizoph.cfm.

National Institute of Mental Health. (2001). *Facts about post-traumatic stress disorder.* Retrieved December 10, 2002, from http://www.nimh.nih.gov/anxiety/ptsdfacts.cfm.

National Resource Center on Homelessness and Mental Illness. (n.d.). *Get the facts: Who is homeless?* Retrieved December 10, 2002, from http://www.nrchmi.com/facts/facts_question_2.asp.

Neistadt, M. E., & Crepeau, E. B. (1998). *Willard & Spackman's occupational therapy* (9th ed.). Philadelphia: Lippincott.

Nelson, C. A. (1995). Cerebral palsy. In D. A. Umphred (Ed.), *Neurological rehabilitation* (3rd ed., pp. 263–286). St. Louis, MO: Mosby.

Newman, E. M., Echevarria, M. E., & Digman, G. (1995). Degenerative diseases. In C. A. Trombly (Ed.), *Occupational therapy for physical dysfunction* (4th ed., pp. 735–741). Baltimore: Williams & Wilkins.

O'Dell, M. W., & Dillon, M. E. (1996). Rehabilitation management in persons with AIDS and HIV infection. In R. L. Braddom, R. M. Buschbacher, D. Dumitru, E. W. Johnson, D. J. Matthews, & M. Sinaki (Eds.), *Physical medicine and rehabilitation.* Philadelphia: W. B. Saunders.

Office for Civil Rights. (1988). *Free appropriate public education for students with handicaps: Requirements under Section 504 of the Rehabilitation Act of 1973.* Washington, DC: Author.

Post Traumatic Stress Disorder Alliance. (n.d.). *What is PTSD?* Retrieved December 10, 2002, from http://www.ptsdalliance.org/about_what.html.

Rancho Los Amigos Medical Center. (1980). *Levels of cognitive functioning.* Downey, CA: Author, Adult Brain Injury Service.

Reed, K. L. (2001). *Quick reference to occupational therapy* (2nd ed.). Gaithersburg, MD: Aspen.

Rock, L. M. (1996). Upper extremity amputations and prosthetics, section 1: Amputations and body powered prostheses. In L. W.

Pedretti (Ed.), *Occupational therapy: Practice skills for physical dysfunction* (4th ed., pp. 567-585). St. Louis, MO: Mosby.

Seibens, H. (1990). Deconditioning. In B. Kemp, K. Brummel-Smith, & J.W. Ramsdell (Eds.), *Geriatric rehabilitation.* Boston: Little, Brown.

South Shore Educational Collaborative. (n.d.). *OT Edge: Sensory Integration.* Retrieved December 11, 2002, from http://www.ssec.org/idis/sseccp/SI.htm.

Stevens, J. R. (1997). Anatomy of schizophrenia revisited. *Schizophrenia Bulletin, 23,* 373-383.

Stolp-Smith, K.A. (1996). Electrodiagnostic medicine III: Case studies. In R. L. Braddom, R. M. Buschbacher, D. Dumitru, E. W. Johnson, D. J. Matthews, & M. Sinaki (Eds.), *Physical medicine and rehabilitation.* Philadelphia: W. B. Saunders.

Tomchek, S. D. (1999). The musculoskeletal system—arthrogryphosis multiplex. In S. M. Poor & E. B. Rainville (Eds.), *Pediatric therapy: A systems approach.* Philadelphia: F.A. Davis.

Tomchek, S. D. (1999). The musculoskeletal system—muscular dystrophy. In S. M. Porr & E. B. Rainville (Eds.), *Pediatric therapy: A systems approach.* Philadelphia: F.A. Davis.

Tooth, L., & McKenna, K. (1996). Contemporary issues in cardiac rehabilitation: Implications for therapists. *British Journal of Occupational Therapy, 59*(3), 133-140.

Turk, D. C., & Melzack, R. (1992). The measurement of pain and the assessment of people experiencing pain. In D. C. Turk & R. Melzack (Eds.), *Handbook of pain assessment.* New York: Guilford Press.

Turk, D. C., Meichenbaum, D., & Genest, M. (1983). *Pain and behavioral medicine.* New York: Guilford Press.

Warren, M. (1998). *Occupational therapy practice guidelines for adults with low vision.* Bethesda, MD: American Occupational Therapy Association.

Weber, R. J., & Lebdusca, S. (1996). Rehabilitation issues in plexopathy. In R. L. Braddom, R. M. Buschbacher, D. Dumitru, E. W. Johnson, D. J. Matthews, & M. Sinaki (Eds.), *Physical medicine and rehabilitation.* Philadelphia: W. B. Saunders.

Williamson, G. G. (1987). *Children with spina bifida.* Baltimore: Paul H. Brookes.

Wilson, D. J., Hickey, K. M., Gorham, J. L., & Childers, M. K. (1997). Lumbar spinal moments in chronic back pain patients during supported lifting: A dynamic analysis. *Archives of Physical Medicine and Rehabilitation, 78,* 967–972.

Winkler, P. (1995). Head injury. In D. A. Humphred (Ed.), *Neurological rehabilitation* (pp. 421–453). St. Louis, MO: Mosby.

Wolinsky, F. D., Fitzgerald, J. F., & Stump, T. E. (1997). The effect of hip fracture on mortality, hospitalization, and functional status: A prospective study. *American Journal of Public Health, 87,* 398–403.

Yarkony, G. M., & Chen, D. (1996). Rehabilitation of patients with spinal cord injuries. In R. L. Braddom, R. Buschbacher, D. Dumitru, E. W. Johnson, D. Matthews, & M. Sinaki (Eds.), *Physical medicine and rehabilitation.* Philadelphia: W. B. Saunders.

Zasler, N. D., Murphy, K., & Holiday, A. (1994). Neurorehabilitation following mild traumatic brain injury. *Rehabilitation Management, 7*(3), 121–123.

Zuckerman, B. (1996). Drug effects: A search for outcomes. *NIDA Research Monograph, 164,* 277–287.